MW01065770

POCKET MANUAL OF
Basic Surgical Skills

POCKET MANUAL OF
Basic Surgical Skills

CHARLES W. VAN WAY III, M.D.

Associate Professor of Surgery,
Department of Surgery,
University of Colorado Health Sciences Center
Denver, Colorado

CHARLES A. BUERK, M.D.

Professor and Chairman,
Department of Surgery,
University of Nevada School of Medicine
Las Vegas, Nevada

With 192 illustrations by

F. Dennis Giddings, A.M.I.

The C. V. Mosby Company

ST. LOUIS • WASHINGTON, D.C. • TORONTO   1986

MOSBY

A TRADITION OF PUBLISHING EXCELLENCE

Editor: Karen Berger
Assistant editor: Ellen Baker Geisel
Project editor: Carlotta Seely
Editing/Production: Kathleen L. Teal
Book design: Gail Morey Hudson

Copyright © 1986 by The C.V. Mosby Company

All rights reserved. No part of this publication may be reproduced, stored in a retrieval system, or transmitted, in any form or by any means, electronic, mechanical, photocopying, recording, or otherwise, without prior written permission from the publisher.

Printed in the United States of America

The C.V. Mosby Company
11830 Westline Industrial Drive, St. Louis, Missouri 63146

Library of Congress Cataloging-in-Publication Data

Van Way, Charles W.
  Pocket manual of basic surgical skills.

  Includes index.
    1. Surgery, Operative—Handbooks, manuals, etc.
2. Surgery—Handbooks, manuals, etc. I. Buerk,
Charles A., 1937—   II. Title. III. Title:
Basic surgical skills.
RD32.V34   1986   617'.91   86-12862
ISBN 0-8016-5231-6

AC/D/D   9 8 7 6 5 4   02/B/292

Foreword

Surgeons formerly held a virtual monopoly on performing operations, and they alone were concerned with operative skills. Along with so many facets of clinical medicine, all this has now changed. Cardiologists routinely perform cut downs on brachial and femoral arteries and make vascular repairs. So do invasive radiologists, who prove their "manipulative" skills by wearing operating room "greens" in the hospital corridors. Dermatologists, oncologists, pediatricians, intensivists, emergency room physicians, and essentially every type of primary physician, regardless of professional roots, suture lacerations, perform needle and excisional biopsies, and introduce central venous or Swan-Ganz catheters.

As long as these various specialists train themselves in the basic performance of such previously "surgical" procedures, there is little evidence that this diffusion of responsibility is detrimental to patient care. However, those who assume responsibility for performing such manipulative procedures must take an equal responsibility for learning these surgical skills—which is what this book is all about.

Surgical Skills in Patient Care (1978) was intended to help medical students in their sophomore course in operative surgery. However, both the course and the experimental laboratories have largely disappeared from most medical schools. Anachronistically, this educational trend has occurred at a time when an increasing number of students, regardless of future specialty, will in subsequent practice require expertise with surgical skills. This pocket manual should be of interest to both students and other clinicians who are assuming the moral and legal responsibility for performing manipulative clinical procedures, whether for diagnosis, monitoring, or treatment.

This manual describes procedures that are either new or have become more frequent in the eight years since the publication of *Surgical Skills in Patient Care*. It includes techniques for introducing central venous pressure lines, newer procedures for Swan-Ganz catheterization, and the burgeoning field of needle and aspiration biopsy of tumors. The final chapter, *Principles of Trauma Care*, reflects the important program sponsored by the American College of Surgeons.

This pocket manual will be invaluable to medical students, junior surgical residents, and an ever-growing number of non-surgical clinicians who are involved in "hands on" clinical practice.

B. Eiseman, M.D.

Denver, Colorado

Foreword to
Surgical Skills in Patient Care

Most medical schools categorize their curricula according to two general headings: knowledge and skills. Like love and successful marriage, the two are inseparable. For example, a bright student may understand all the essentials of wound healing; however, if he lacks the ability to place sutures or to tie knots, this knowledge, alone, becomes meaningless to the patient with a laceration.

Similarly, although we live in an era of specialization, critically ill patients cannot always wait for a specialist to insert an endotracheal tube or an intravenous line, or to perform defibrillation of the heart. Any professional who takes care of patients should become adept at these elemental techniques.

The authors have had a rich experience in teaching these skills to residents, medical students, and other medical personnel. From this background they have selected certain procedures that they believe to be basic to the care of patients—procedures that all who take responsibility for patients should know.

In this manual, concise instructions illustrated by drawings will help students gain confidence as they begin to perform these procedures and will reinforce this confidence as they learn that these techniques are based on solid clinical experience.

I believe that all who become familiar with this book will agree with the University of Colorado housestaff and students that Doctors Buerk and Van Way present these important skills in an especially adept way.

R.D. Liechty, M.D.

Professor of Surgery
University of Colorado Medical Center
Denver, Colorado

Preface

This book is a "first edition" in the new *Pocket Manual* series. It is actually a revision of our earlier text, *Surgical Skills in Patient Care*. This text was written from our experience in teaching basic surgical technique to medical students.

Medical progress has made us all surgeons. Every physician must do some—or all—of the procedures described in this text. Such specialties as emergency medicine, cardiology, and invasive radiology may require a considerable range of surgical skills.

Pocket Manual of Basic Surgical Skills is directed toward three groups. First, medical students, who must cope with an increasingly technique-oriented body of medical knowledge, and yet who are usually given no formal course in surgical skills. Second, the young surgeon in training, who has our sympathy. Finally, and perhaps most important, the nonsurgical specialist, who has no surgical training, and yet who must do these procedures daily.

This is a personal text. Both of us are active general surgeons, and we have drawn heavily from our own experiences in performing these techniques. Every procedure described has been done by one or both of us, and the techniques are those which we have found to be the best. Where relevant, we have explained our rationale. We make no apologies to those who do this procedure or that in a different way. But recognizing that there is more than one path to virtue, we claim no exclusive right to surgical truth. If another technique works, use it.

Charles W. Van Way III, M.D.
Charles A. Buerk, M.D.

Contents

1

Aseptic technique

Medicine has advanced further in the last 100 years than in all the preceding years. The most important component of that advance is the ability to manipulate or operate on the human body without fear of infection. This ability makes possible intravenous therapy, invasive diagnostic procedures, injection of drugs, care of wounds, and the entire field of operative surgery. The basis for this ability is the group of techniques known collectively as *aseptic*, or *sterile, technique.*

The terms *aseptic* and *sterile* are often used interchangeably. The distinction between them is subtle. *Aseptic* refers to the complete absence of living microorganisms, as might be produced by autoclaving an instrument pack. *Sterile* also means the absence of living microorganisms, but this state may be produced by chemical agents, as in preparation of the skin through which an operation is to be performed. Originally, sterile technique was carried out entirely with chemicals such as carbolic acid (phenol), which were used on instruments and on the skin. This was known as *antiseptic technique.* With the introduction of the steam autoclave and other physical techniques more effective than chemicals in sterilizing instruments and linens, the term *aseptic technique* was used to distinguish the newer methods from the older chemical methods. However, distinction has been lost. Current aseptic technique relies on both chemical and physical methods for achieving sterility.

Aseptic technique is based on the premise that infection is introduced into the body from outside. To avoid infection it is necessary to ensure that any procedure performed on the body is done in such a way as to introduce no bacteria. The procedure must be done in a sterile field from which all living bacteria have been excluded, including those initially present on the patient's skin. All instruments, sutures, and fluids must be sterilized. The surgeon's hands must be cleansed of all bacteria and encased in rubber gloves, or the procedure must be done without the surgeon's hands touching the sterile end of the instruments.

The principles of aseptic care are no less important in minor procedures than in major operations. Sepsis associated with a venous cutdown can kill just as surely as infection introduced at the operating table. This chapter outlines the methods of preparing the skin, washing the hands, sterilizing instruments and fluids, and setting up the sterile field in which all procedures must be done.

SKIN PREPARATION

Bacteria are normally present on the skin. It is necessary both to clean all dirt from the skin and to sterilize the skin with some form of antiseptic solution. Several antiseptics have been used over the years.

Iodine is one of the oldest antiseptics still in use. Although iodine is an excellent antiseptic, it is also somewhat toxic and may burn the skin. If iodine is used, the skin should be cleaned off immediately with alcohol.

The iodophors are a group of compounds in which iodine is combined with an organic molecule. They are available as detergent-containing solutions for washing the hands and as nondetergent "prep" solutions for preparing the skin. The iodine is released from its organic complex slowly enough to avoid burning the skin but rapidly enough to kill bacteria. In the operating room the skin is usually cleansed first with the detergent solution to remove dirt and oils. After the skin is dried, the nondetergent solution is painted on, with a thin film of iodophor left on the skin.

Alcohol is widely used in preparing the skin for venipuncture and intramuscular injections. Although alcohol cleans the skin, it inadequately kills bacteria. Isopropyl alcohol and ethanol are equally ineffective. Therefore the practice of swabbing the skin before an injection is probably unnecessary.

Mercury is an effective antiseptic. Mercuric chloride is toxic to the skin. Merbromin (Mercurochrome) is widely used as an antiseptic but is ineffective. More effective are the organic mercurial compounds, of which thimerosal (Merthiolate) is the most widely used. These compounds are relatively nontoxic but penetrate skin poorly; they are bacteriostatic rather than bactericidal. They do not kill spores, and skin sensitization may occur.

Ordinary detergent soap solutions do not kill bacteria, but detergent solution with hexachlorophene (pHisoHex) is often used. Hexachlorophene is a phenol with a mild antibacterial effect that is cumulative; if it is used three or four times daily, the bacterial count on the skin is reduced significantly. Hexachlorophene is often used as a surgical scrub solution.

Chlorhexidine gluconate (Hibiclens) is widely used. Chemically, it is hexamethylene-bis-biguanide in 4% isopropyl alcohol, and soap. It is bactericidal with persisting antimicrobial activity. Since chlorhexidine gluconate is nonirritating, it is commonly used for hand preparation and for the operation site.

Certain cationic surface-active agents are used in skin preparation; the most common is benzalkonium chloride (Zephiran). These agents are bactericidal and relatively fast acting but slower acting than iodine. They have detergent action and penetrate tissue surfaces; but they are antagonized by soap, pus, and tissue fluids. On the skin these agents tend to form a film under which bacteria may remain. Because of their relatively low toxicity, they may be used on sensitive areas, such as the eye or the mucous membranes, where iodophors might be harmful.

In preparing an operative field, the usual principle is to begin at the center and work outward (Fig. 1-1). An exception should

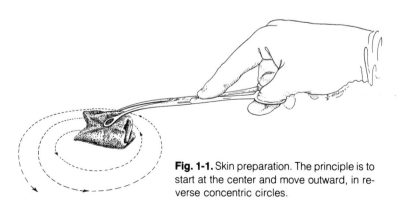

Fig. 1-1. Skin preparation. The principle is to start at the center and move outward, in reverse concentric circles.

be made for a contaminated wound: the skin surrounding the wound is prepared first and the wound cleansed last. In all situations the area prepared should be much wider than the proposed operative field.

The time required for adequate skin preparation is 5 minutes. When skin is cleansed with an iodophor-containing detergent, the residual bacterial count will drop markedly during the first minute and progressively less during the second and third minutes. After 5 minutes the count will be minimal. Further skin preparation is nonproductive, although many operating rooms use a routine 10-minute scrub of the operative field.

HAND PREPARATION

Although the surgeon's hands are covered with sterile gloves, they must be scrubbed. The surgeon's hands may carry pathogenic bacteria acquired from other patients. Gloves often become punctured or torn during the procedure. Even without gross tears, small unsuspected punctures often occur.

Iodophor, hexachlorophene, and chlorhexidine gluconate are all commonly used for this purpose. They are mixed with detergent to give a cleansing action along with the antibacterial action. Disposable, presterilized scrub sponges impregnated with one of these agents are available. Iodophors and chlorhexidine are much more effective for one-time use. Detergent solutions containing hexachlorophene are little more effective than detergent alone on first use. However, the hexachlorophene accumulates on the epidermis of the surgeon's hands and after 2 to 4 days of habitual use reduces the bacterial count to 5% or less of the initial value. Because of this, hexachlorophene is widely used by surgeons. To be effective it must be used regularly, several times a day.

In standard scrub technique the hands are first mechanically cleansed (Fig. 1-2). Particular attention should be paid to the nails. Any visible dirt under the nails should be removed by vigorous brushing or by a nail file or a plastic nail pick. Then a 5-minute scrub should be carried out, beginning at the fingers and working meticulously up the hand and forearm to the elbows. Although some operating rooms specify a 10-minute scrub, 5 minutes is enough.

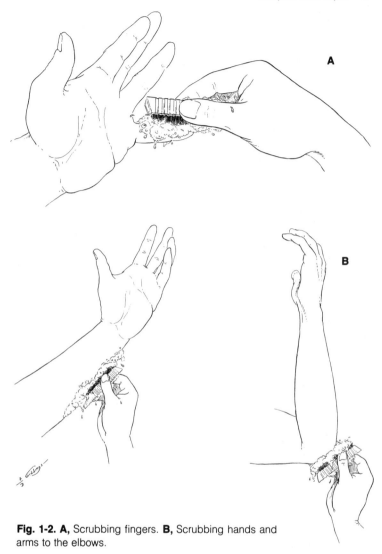

Fig. 1-2. A, Scrubbing fingers. **B,** Scrubbing hands and arms to the elbows.

After the hands are dried and the gloves put on, the hands usually begin to sweat. Bacteria are washed from deep pores up onto the surface of the skin. Even if an iodophor detergent solution is used, the bacterial count rises nearly to initial values after an hour or so. There is no justification to the practice of "saving" the scrub by keeping gown and gloves on between cases. If hexachlorophene solutions have been used habitually, the bacterial count will remain low. A surgeon using hexachlorophene routinely can reduce the scrub between cases from 5 minutes to 3 minutes.

Although the surgical scrub is primarily applicable to the operating room, all but the most minor procedures should be preceded by scrubbing the hands. It is discouraging to watch physicians roll up their sleeves, put on a pair of gloves, and proceed to place a tube in the chest or a biopsy needle in the liver without first washing their hands.

TECHNIQUES OF STERILIZATION

Five techniques are commonly used for sterilizing instruments and fluids: steam autoclaving, ethylene oxide sterilization, soaking in germicidal solutions, irradiation, and Millipore filtration of solutions.

Steam autoclaving is used for preparing instrument packs in the operating room and in central supply areas. The use of steam under pressure allows for temperatures above that of boiling water; the steam is necessary to allow the heat to penetrate wrapped instrument packs. Generally, a temperature of approximately 120° C (250° F) with a pressure of 20 to 25 pounds is used for 15 to 30 minutes. Unwrapped metal instruments require only 15 minutes of sterilization, but wrapped linen packs require about 30 minutes. Tape or other indicators that change color after exposure to heat are used as a check on whether or not enough heat has been applied. However, such indicators are not infallible. For example, steam will not penetrate between the jaws of a closed clamp. Steam also will not penetrate small caliber needles, unless a stylet or small wire is placed inside the needle.

Ethylene oxide is a germicidal gas that sterilizes at the relatively low temperature range of 50° to 60° C (120° to 150° F). It is widely used for instruments that would be damaged by heat. The gas is toxic and must be used in a specially designed autoclave. An exposure of 3 hours or more is required to kill all bacteria and spores. Sterilization indicators similar to those used in steam sterilization are available. One major disadvantage of the method is that the gas permeates plastics and rubber. All instruments should be allowed to aerate for at least 24 hours before use. If implantable devices such as artificial valves or vascular prostheses are sterilized in this manner, an aeration time of 5 to 7 days should elapse between sterilization and use.

So-called cold sterilization, in which the instruments are soaked in solutions of formalin or iodophors, is widely used for instruments in daily use, such as cystoscopes. This method of sterilization is quite effective, although the instruments must be rinsed carefully.

Most manufacturers of sterile medical devices and intravenous fluids use high-dose gamma irradiation, usually from a cobalt source. This method is used in almost all prepackaged sterile supplies. It is especially suitable for plastics, which would be damaged by the heat of autoclaving. This method is virtually an ideal one, its only disadvantage being the high initial cost of the equipment involved.

In sterilizing fluids in small batches, as in the hospital pharmacy, Millipore filtration is commonly used. In this method the fluid is passed through a 0.22 micron filter, which will not allow any bacteria or spores to pass.

THE STERILE FIELD

In performing a procedure the first step is to establish a sterile field. The instrument pack is opened, the hands are scrubbed

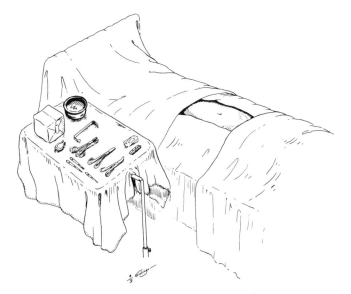

Fig. 1-3. Sterile table and sterile field.

(Fig. 1-2), gloves are put on, and the skin is prepared with a ring forceps or large clamp and sponges (Fig. 1-1). Towels, and sheets if necessary, are placed around the site of the procedure. At this point there is a sterile instrument pack on the table and a sterile operative site surrounded by sterile towels (Fig. 1-3). Anything needed during the procedure must be handed into the sterile field by someone outside it. For this reason it takes a minimum of two people to do most procedures: one with gloved hands, working within the sterile field, and one with nonsterile hands, to pass supplies and instruments into the sterile field. Sterile supplies and needles are always packaged to permit opening by an individual with nonsterile hands who would hand the sterile item into the sterile field.

GOWNS, CAPS, AND MASKS

When carrying out a sterile procedure, the practitioner should always wear a surgical cap and mask. The cap prevents nonsterile material from falling into the sterile field. The classic surgical cap is adequate for men or women with short hair. Long hair requires a more voluminous cap, and a beard calls for the "helmet" type of headgear. Masks come in a variety of shapes and sizes. Their purpose is to prevent droplets of sputum from reaching the sterile field. Both caps and masks are generally made of paper and are disposable.

A gown is worn for extensive or lengthy procedures, or when it is necessary to put the forearms into the field. It is difficult to do much suturing without inadvertently touching the suture material with the forearms. Gloves alone could be used in suturing a minor laceration or performing a cutdown, but a procedure such as a cardiac catheterization or suturing a large laceration would require a gown. Only that portion of a gown that can be easily seen should be considered sterile; this includes the sleeves below the upper arms and the front of the gown above the waist. Although the whole gown is sterile in the beginning, it is easy to brush unknowingly against a nonsterile object with the sides, back, shoulder, or skirt of the gown.

Putting on gloves while wearing a sterile gown is a minor technical feat in itself. The closed technique is universally used (Fig. 1-4). In this technique the hands are kept within the sleeves

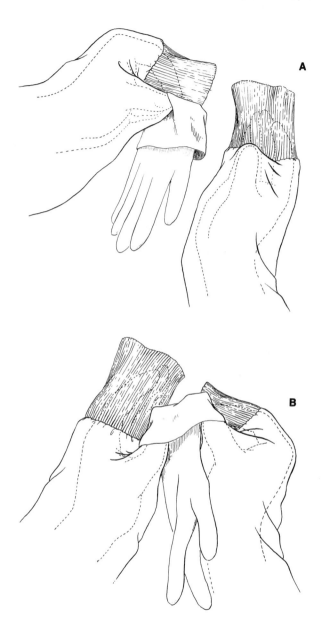

Fig. 1-4. A, Left hand with gown picking up glove. **B,** Left hand putting gown on right sleeve; right thumb grasping through gown.

Continued.

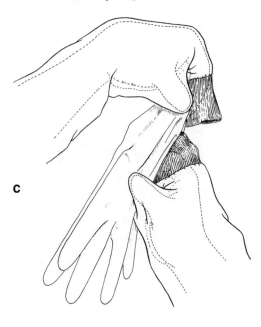

Fig. 1-4, cont'd. C, Left hand (through gown) pulling right glove and sleeve over right hand. **D,** Right hand in glove, sleeve at wrist, and left hand still pulling down.

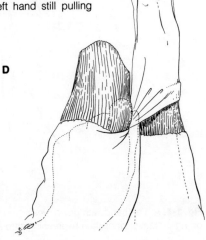

of the gown. A glove is picked up with one covered hand and placed on the end of the other sleeve. The other hand is then advanced into the glove. The second glove is picked up with the gloved hand and placed on the end of the first sleeve. The first hand is then advanced into the glove. This technique is somewhat intricate but is relatively easy to learn. The advantage is that since the bare hand is never advanced beyond the end of the cuff there is no way that it can contaminate the gown or the gloves.

•   •   •

In summary, aseptic technique is a body of techniques for ensuring that all bacteria are excluded from the nonsterile field in which the procedure is to be done. Although the details may vary from procedure to procedure, the basic techniques must be followed in every invasive procedure.

2

The tools of patient care

The instruments used by today's practitioners have evolved over the years as surgeons and physicians have developed new instruments or modified existing ones to meet certain demands and accomplish specific tasks. A knowledge of the basic instruments will greatly facilitate the minor procedures that all physicians and practitioners will be called on to perform. These instruments or minor variations are found in all minor surgery packs.

CUTTING INSTRUMENTS

The disposable scalpel blade attached to a standard handle is used primarily for incising the skin, although some surgeons use it for dissecting deeper tissues. Different sizes and shapes of blades are available for specific purposes, as are different sizes of handles. For most general work a No. 3 handle is used with a No. 10, No. 11, or No. 15 blade (Fig. 2-1).

The No. 10 blade is the most useful disposable blade for making skin incisions. The belly of the blade, not the point, should be used in making the incision. Because the blade is extremely sharp, little pressure is needed in making the incision. The No. 15 blade, a smaller version of the No. 10 blade, is useful in making small incisions or when curved or precise incisions are necessary. Because the belly of this blade is closer to the point, its cutting angle to the skin is increased. Both of these blades should be kept perpendicular to the skin so that there will be no beveling of the skin edges. In using these blades, the handle of the scalpel should be held as depicted in Fig. 2-2. Because of the "flat" belly of the No. 10 blade, it is not usually held like a pencil. When precise work is required, the No. 15 blade can be manipulated as a pencil. The No. 11 blade should be used for incising abscesses and other collections. The blade should be thrust point

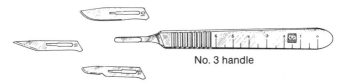

Fig. 2-1. Scalpel handle with three most commonly used disposable scalpel blades.

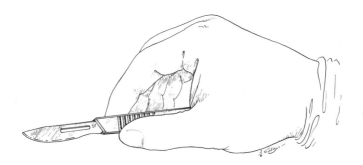

Fig. 2-2. Proper method for holding scalpel.

first into the abscess and withdrawn in a sweeping motion so that the initial incision is enlarged.

Scissors have undegone numerous adaptations over the years, one of which is the development of scissors designed specifically for the cutting of tissues. Typically these scissors have curved blades with a fine cutting edge and rounded points. *Mayo scissors* (Fig. 2-3) are heavy scissors designed for division of tougher structures, such as fascia and tendons, and come with either curved or straight blades. *Metzenbaum scissors* (Fig. 2-4), which are much lighter, are used in dissecting and cutting tissue. For precise, minute dissection, *iris scissors* (Fig. 2-5) are often helpful. Tissue scissors are delicate instruments and should be used only for their designed tasks. They should not be used to cut sutures or bandage material or they will be ruined. Other types of scissors have been designed for these purposes (Fig. 2-6).

All scissors are designed for right-handed use so that when grasped properly, as shown in Fig. 2-7, good shearing is obtained by mild outward pressure of the thumb in conjunction with inward pressure by the fingers. Note that in right-handed use the

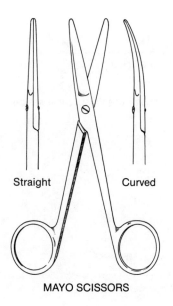

Fig. 2-3

Straight   Curved

MAYO SCISSORS

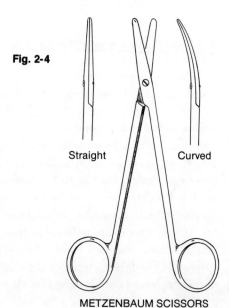

Fig. 2-4

Straight   Curved

METZENBAUM SCISSORS

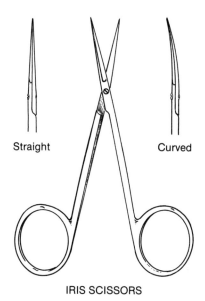

Fig. 2-5

Straight

Curved

IRIS SCISSORS

Fig. 2-6

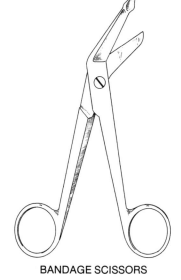

BANDAGE SCISSORS

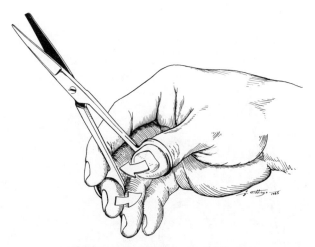

Fig. 2-7. Right-handed use of scissors.

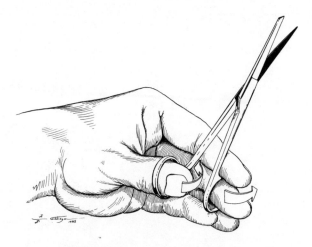

Fig. 2-8. Left-handed use of scissors.

fingers are not inserted into the loops past the first knuckle. During left-handed use, however, the pressure relationships are reversed and a pulling motion of the thumb is employed, which usually requires the insertion of the thumb into the loop past the first knuckle (Fig. 2-8). Left-handed persons learn this naturally, but right-handed persons have difficulty when forced to use their left hand.

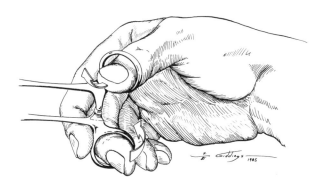

Fig. 2-9. Pressure relationships in right-handed use of ratchet lock forceps.

GRASPING INSTRUMENTS

Thumb forceps (Fig. 2-9) are designed to hold and immobilize tissue during dissection. Forceps with teeth hold tissue well with minimal pressure to prevent slipping, but for obvious reasons these instruments are not used on structures that may be punctured.

The most useful thumb forceps are called *toothed forceps* and are used in grasping and immobilizing subcutaneous tissues, muscle, and fascia during dissection or suturing. A finer toothed forceps, the *Adson forceps,* is particularly useful in skin closure.

Smooth forceps (without teeth) are useful in stabilizing tissues that might be perforated and in holding gauze sponges to clean out wounds. Because more pressure is needed to hold tissue firmly, these forceps are not used to hold the skin.

Grasping forceps are designed to hold tissue firmly enough to allow for traction. Typically they have finger rings and box ratchet locks. The ratchet locks are designed to function with the same pressure relationship as scissors. These locks are handled differently by the right and left hand, as shown in Figs. 2-10 and 2-11. These are basically "right-handed" instruments, as are scissors, and their use is different for the two hands.

Allis and *Kocher forceps* are shown in Fig. 2-12. *Allis forceps* have finely serrated teeth on pliable jaws that limit the amount of

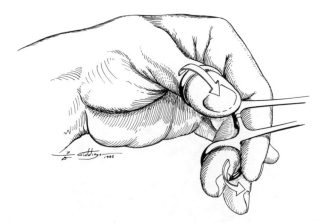

Fig. 2-10. Inverse pressure relationships in left-handed use of ratchet lock forceps.

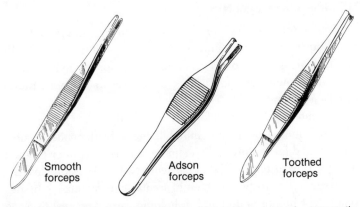

Smooth forceps

Adson forceps

Toothed forceps

Fig. 2-11. Types of thumb forceps: toothed for traction, Adson for atraumatic grasping, and smooth for stabilization.

pressure applied. They are useful for grasping fascia and for holding and removing biopsy material. *Kocher forceps* have three interlocking teeth with strong rigid jaws that can exert considerable pressure. They are used when strong traction is required on tough tissues such as fascia. They are also useful in grasping foreign bodies.

Certain forceps have been developed specifically for the control of bleeding. These *hemostatic forceps* (Fig. 2-13) are similar

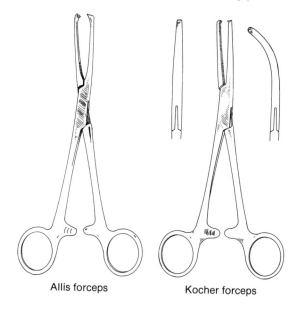

Allis forceps   Kocher forceps

Fig. 2-12

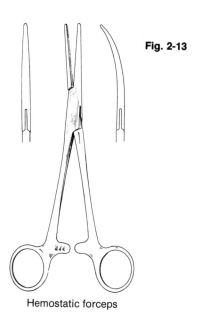

Fig. 2-13

Hemostatic forceps

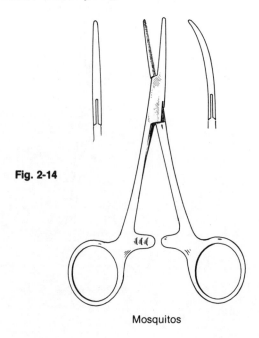

Fig. 2-14

Mosquitos

to grasping forceps, having finger rings and box ratchet locks, but they have finer jaws for more precise application. Although these are identified by numerous eponyms with regional preferences, *hemostat, stat,* or *snap* will suffice. For general use, they are 5 to 6 inches in length and have either curved or straight jaws. Smaller, more delicate instruments are called *mosquitos* (Fig. 2-14) and are used when even more precise application is required. In applying hemostatic forceps, only the minimal amount of tissue is grasped, since subsequent application of the ligature will cause tissue necrosis. Only the points of the forceps should be used to minimize the inclusion of extraneous tissue. The practitioner should try to avoid putting fingers far into the rings because when trying to extricate the fingers it is easy to tear the small amount of tissue held in the clamp.

Needle holders (Fig. 2-15) are also modifications of the basic grasping forceps. These instruments typically have stronger, shorter, and wider jaws than hemostats so that considerable pressure can be applied to the needle. The needle is grasped one half to three quarters of the way from the point, with the point protruding to the left (in right-handed operators), so that pronation

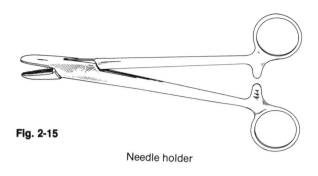

Fig. 2-15

Needle holder

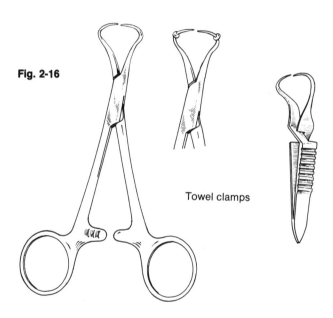

Fig. 2-16

Towel clamps

will drive the needle through the tissue in the desired arc. Learning to tie with the needle holder (see Chapter 3; Technique IV) will facilitate many procedures.

Ring forceps are usually used with gauze sponges to clean out the wound or prepare the skin. *Towel clamps* (Fig. 2-16) are used to secure the sterile towels around the operative area.

RETRACTING INSTRUMENTS

Retractors are helpful in holding tissue out of the way and providing adequate exposure. Although many types of retractors

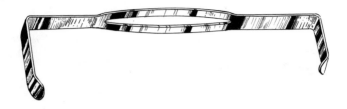

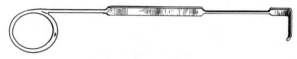

Smooth manual retractors

Fig. 2-17

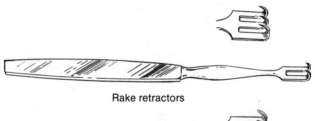

Rake retractors

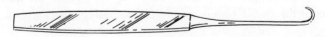

Skin hook

Fig. 2-18

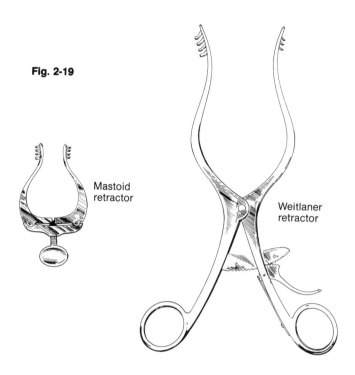

Fig. 2-19

Mastoid retractor

Weitlaner retractor

have been developed, the practitioner need be acquainted with only a few of the most important ones.

Manual retractors can be considered extensions of the hand. Smooth retractors, such as the *Army-Navy* and *finger retractors* (Fig. 2-17), are designed primarily for providing exposure in deeper wounds. The blunt-toothed *rake retractor* (Fig. 2-18) is beneficial in applying traction to subcutaneous tissue and muscle, where there is little danger of perforating a blood vessel or viscus. The *skin hook* and *sharp rake* provide effective means of immobilizing or retracting skin edges.

Self-retaining retractors (Fig. 2-19) have blades that are applied to both edges of the wound and then spread apart. They have a locking mechanism that holds the blades open. This frees the practitioner and the assistant for other tasks. The *mastoid* and *Weitlaner* retractors are useful for small incisions and provide satisfactory retraction of superficial tissues. Numerous modifications of this type of retractor exist.

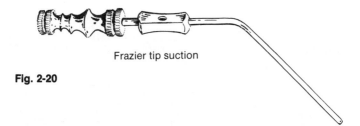

Frazier tip suction

Fig. 2-20

SUCTION DEVICES

It is often necessary, even in minor procedures, to remove blood for adequate visualization. This can usually be accomplished by swabbing the wound with gauze sponges. In some instances brisk bleeding may require suctioning. The best suction apparatus for minor procedures is the *Frazier tip suction* (Fig. 2-20). The thumb vent on this instrument allows the operator to break the suction at the tip so that tissue is not aspirated into the metal tube.

ELECTROSURGICAL APPARATUS

In the 1920s neurosurgeon Harvey Cushing collaborated with an electrical engineer, William Bovie, to produce a device that used radio frequency electric current to coagulate bleeding vessels. Their original device used a modified spark gap radio transmitter to generate the coagulation current. Subsequently, electrosurgical apparatus has gone through three generations of refinements, first with vacuum tubes, then transistors, and, most recently, microprocessor controlled circuits. Electrosurgical devices are used in all operating rooms and are frequently found in outpatient clinics and physicians' offices.

The basic principle is that continuous high frequency (HF) electrical current cuts tissue (Fig. 2-21). If the current is interrupted and the energy concentrated in short "packets," coagulation is produced. "Blended cutting" is a combination of the two. A typical frequency would be 500 kilohertz (500,000 cycles per second). A typical interruption rate would be 20 kilohertz. There are more exotic forms of electrosurgery, such as "spray mode" or "ion beam" coagulation, but these are simply modifications of the basic principle.

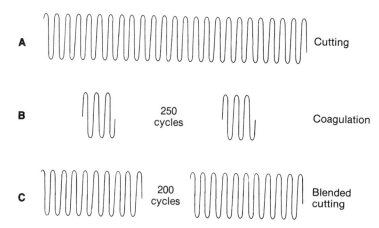

Fig. 2-21. Wave forms of electrocoagulation. **A,** Pure cutting. **B,** Pure coagulation. Actually this will cut the power if set high enough. **C,** Blended cutting. The shorter the burst of energy, the greater the coagulation effect relative to the cutting effect.

Power levels range from 10 to 250 watts, depending on the machine and its settings. Most work is done in the 20- to 80-watt range. Note the effect of the wave form in Fig. 2-21. For a given power level, the instantaneous power, "watts per cycle," is much higher for coagulation than for cutting because the same amount of energy is carried in fewer cycles.

The actual mechanism of cutting and coagulation remains somewhat obscure. The effect of the cutting current appears to be caused by local vaporization of tissue by the continuous wave. The coagulation current, occurring in small high-intensity bursts, allows the tissue to cool off between bursts of energy. Coagulation, rather than vaporization, is produced. Although it is tempting to assume that the effect is largely the result of heat production, replacing the electrosurgical pencil with a hot iron cautery does not produce the same kind of cutting or coagulation. Electrosurgical cutting and coagulation appears to be much more localized than hot iron coagulation and is much more selective in its action. For example, radio frequency current travels preferentially down blood vessels because of the low impedance of the blood. There is selective coagulation of blood vessels, an obvious aid to hemostasis.

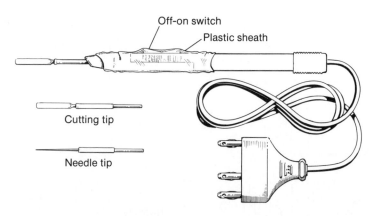

Off-on switch

Plastic sheath

Cutting tip

Needle tip

Fig. 2-22. Electrosurgical tools.

The tool of electrosurgery is the electrosurgical pencil, with a ball, cutting, or needle tip electrode (Fig. 2-22). The electrosurgical pencil generally has a switch to allow turning on either the cutting current or the coagulation current. In older units this may be accomplished with a foot switch. Using an electrosurgical pencil requires a somewhat different touch than using a knife. For one thing, this tool should be gripped like a pencil. Most electrosurgical pencils have the switch located a little too far back for comfort. A certain amount of contortion of the hand may be necessary to comfortably work the switch and at the same time apply the blade to tissue. Electrosurgical cutting is not generally used on the skin, since dividing the epidermis by electrosurgery allegedly leaves a thicker and more prominent scar than cutting it with a knife. However, there is some question as to whether this is true for the more modern electrosurgical generators. The effect of electrosurgical cutting is somewhat like using an extremely sharp knife. As the blade moves, the tissue should part almost without resistance. A certain amount of carbonization on the blade occurs with both cutting and coagulation, and it is necessary to clean the blade periodically.

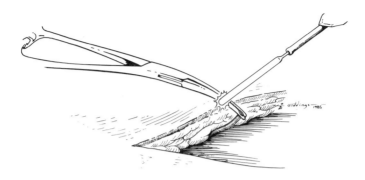

Fig. 2-23. Applying electrosurgical current.

The technique of electrocoagulation generally involves placing a clamp on the blood vessel and applying the electrosurgical current to the clamp (Fig. 2-23). Alternatively the blood may be dried and electrosurgical current applied directly to the tissue. This works better with the new spray mode or the still newer ion beam coagulator than with more conventional electrocoagulation.

The machine should be set to provide a power level just sufficient to do the work that needs to be done. Excess power may cause damage.

There is an ongoing debate over the relative damage produced by electrosurgical dissection and by conventional (knife and suture) dissection. The best evidence to date indicates that cutting with the electrosurgical current produces somewhat more tissue damage than cutting with the knife. Coagulation with electrosurgery, however, produces no more damage than suture control of bleeding and may produce less.

3

Sutures, needles, and knot tying

A bewildering variety of sutures and needles are available to the surgeon (see box). Although the choice of suture and needle is often arbitrary, certain principles are observed. Usually, any of several sutures and needles is satisfactory for a given task.

SUTURE MATERIALS

There are two basic kinds of suture: absorbable and nonabsorbable. The absorbable sutures are plain gut, chromic gut, polyglycolic acid, polyglactin, and polydioxanone. An inflammatory reaction will cause the suture material to be absorbed by the body after several weeks. Therefore it follows that all absorbable sutures will produce some degree of tissue reaction.

Absorbable sutures

Plain and *chromic gut* sutures are produced from the tough submucosal layer of hog intestine. The plain gut suture is unmodified and will lose tensile strength in 1 to 2 weeks. The chromic gut suture is soaked in chromic acid salts, which are the same compounds used for tanning leather. This process results in a suture that usually retains its strength for 2 to 3 weeks. Both sutures are damaged by drying and therefore are packaged wet.

Since gut suture material is stiff, hard to tie, and causes a great deal of tissue reaction, it is not a good choice. Also with the introduction of polyglycolic acid and polyglactin 910, gut is being superseded.

Dexon, which is *polyglycolic acid*, and *Vicryl*, which is *polyglactin 910*, are both synthetic. These sutures retain their strength for 2 to 3 weeks, and their behavior is somewhat more predictable. The inflammatory reaction is not as marked as in plain and chromic gut sutures. Polyglactin 910 is absorbed slightly more rapidly than polyglycolic acid. Complete absorption for

SUTURES

ABSORBABLE SUTURES
Plain gut
Chromic gut
Dexon (polyglycolic acid, Davis & Geck)
Vicryl (polyglactin 910, Ethicon)
Polydioxanone (PDS, Ethicon)

NONABSORBABLE SUTURES
Silk
Twisted or braided

Cotton
Twisted

Dacron Polyester
Braided
    Dacron (Deknatel, Davis & Geck)
    Mersilene (Ethicon)
Braided, impregnated with Teflon
    Ethiflex (Ethicon)
    Tevdek (Deknatel; heavily impregnated)
    Polydek (Deknatel; lightly impregnated)
Braided, treated with silicone
    Ti-cron (Davis & Geck)
Braided, coated with polybutilate
    Ethibond (Ethicon)

Nylon
Monofilament
Braided (Nurolon, Ethicon; Surgilene, Davis & Geck, Surgical nylon, Deknotel)

Polypropylene
Monofilament (Prolene, Ethicon; Surgilene, Davis & Geck)

Stainless steel
Monofilament
Braided (Flexon, Davis & Geck, Deklene, Deknatel, Braided steel, Ethicon)

polyglactin 910 is reached at 80 days, and for polyglycolic acid at 120 days. Chromic gut is absorbed somewhat faster, reaching 90% absorption at 50 days and complete absorption at 80 days.

PDS, which is *polydioxanone*, is a monofilament synthetic absorbable suture. It retains its strength for 4 to 6 weeks (50% at 4 weeks) and is completely absorbed within 6 months. Since it is a monofilament, it is especially useful in suturing infected or contaminated wounds.

Nonabsorbable sutures

The nonabsorbable sutures can be divided into four groups: silk and cotton, braided synthetics, monofilament synthetics, and wire. *Silk* and *cotton* are, of course, the oldest. Silk is the most widely used, but it is not, strictly speaking, nonabsorbable. Silk loses its tensile strength progressively over about a year, and it is absorbed by the end of 2 years. It elicits more inflammatory reaction than any of the other nonabsorbable sutures, but it is easy to handle and tie.

The *braided synthetic* sutures consist of several types: polyester, polyester impregnated with Teflon in varying degrees, and nylon. There are a number of brand names for each, as indicated on p. 29. All of the braided synthetics are considerably less reactive than silk, but silk holds knots well and will stay securely tied with three half-knots. Most of the synthetics require five or six half-knots for an equal degree of security. They also require more time and effort to tie and more suture material is left in the wound. Because of this, silk is commonly used for ligating vessels, and is still widely used for sutures.

Braided synthetic sutures are usually made of Dacron polyester. Dacron is a brand name for a DuPont polymer fiber. It may be unmodified, impregnated with Teflon, or treated with silicone or polybutilate. Nylon braided suture is also available.

There is a continuous debate over synthetics vs silk. The braided synthetics share the advantage of being less reactive than silk, and most are stronger than silk for a given size. This is not necessarily important; if tensile strength is desired, a larger silk suture could be substituted with little disadvantage. Synthetic material is more expensive than silk, but packaging and needle costs are so large a part of the total cost that this is not a great disadvantage. Silk elicits more inflammation than the synthetic sutures.

Each of the three major suture manufacturers produces its own particular kinds of braided synthetic sutures. Although the basic materials are the same, there are real differences among the products. Tying and knot-holding properties vary considerably with the method of manufacture. For example, sutures heavily impregnated with Teflon do not hold knots as well as unimpregnated polyester sutures. All of the synthetic sutures have good retention of tensile strength over many years. All multiple-strand sutures (including silk, cotton, polyester, and braided wire) share the drawback of harboring bacteria within the suture. In infected wounds they tend to protect the bacteria from attack by the body's defenses. Characteristically, an infected suture is encysted by the body in small abscess form, and if left undisturbed, will eventually work its way out to the skin. An infected wound will "spit" sutures for a year or more.

Teflon impregnation is used in an attempt to decrease the tendency of braided suture to perpetuate an infection. The theory is that the Teflon fills the interstices, leaving no room for bacteria. Unfortunately, this theory does not work well in practice. In the infected wound, sutures heavily impregnated with Teflon do not appear to be as inert as monofilament sutures although they may be better than unmodified polyester. Teflon impregnation adversely affects ease of handling and knot tying.

The *monofilament sutures*, polypropylene and nylon, are the most inert. They are somewhat more difficult to handle and tie and hold knots poorly. Nylon is worse than polypropylene. Polypropylene is a softer material and, assuming good technique is used in tying the knots, will hold knots nearly as well as braided polyester suture. The monofilament sutures are inert and do not tend to harbor bacteria. In an infected wound they are more likely to heal without stitch abscesses. They also hold their strength well with time.

Wire sutures are made of very high grade stainless steel, since ordinary steel would corrode in the body. Stainless steel is available both as a monofilament and as a braided suture. In theory monofilament wire is as inert as the monofilament sutures, although in practice this is not so. Wire sutures adapt to tissue poorly, resulting in small open spaces around the suture, and for this reason wire has no advantage in infected wounds. Wire is extremely difficult to tie, and the larger sizes must be twisted rather than tied. However, this is an advantage when suturing bone, because the suture can be twisted down to the desired degree of tension. For example, it is often used in closing sternotomy wounds. Wire retains its strength well for a long time.

SUTURE SIZES

The classic suture sizes were taken from thread sizes available when sutures were simply sewing thread. The sizing method is cumbersome but well established. The largest suture available is No. 5, which is approximately the size of ordinary string. The sizes are numbered progressively down to No. 1, which is still a heavy suture. Below this, suture sizes begin with 0 and progress downward through 00, 000, 4-0, to 10-0. For ordinary use, 4-0 through 0 are standard. No. 5-0 through 7-0 sutures are used for delicate vascular anastomoses and 8-0 through 10-0 for microvascular work and eye surgery. Sizes 0 and 1 are suitable for heavy fascial repair, and sizes 2 through 5 are used mostly for bones and tendons. In comparison, a strand of human hair would be the same size as a 6-0 to 7-0 suture.

SUTURE CHOICES

The first thing to decide is whether to use absorbable or nonabsorbable suture. The basic principle is to use an absorbable suture where continued strength is not important, or when infection would make it desirable for the suture to be absorbed. Nonabsorbable suture is used when tissue reaction should be minimal, when continued strength is desirable, or when the suture will be removed subsequently. Nonabsorbable suture is used in the skin and in fascial closure. Absorbable suture is generally used for the subcutaneous tissue and the mucosal layer of the intestine. Often, either one will do, such as in ligating small vessels.

When getting down to the finer points, the choice of suture becomes a matter of opinion. In a similar situation one surgeon may use chromic gut, another might choose Dexon, and still another might use silk. Most surgeons use either polypropylene or monofilament nylon in the skin. These sutures are the most inert and have the least reaction around their entry site; therefore they leave the least scar. Silk is generally considered too reactive for the skin, except for wounds from which the sutures will be removed in 2 or 3 days. Some orthopedic surgeons use an intracuticular suture of monofilament wire whose strength allows it to be pulled out later. Many surgeons close skin with a 4-0 Dexon intracuticular suture.

Staples (AutoSuture or Ethicon) are often used on the skin. Even though they are expensive, they can be rapidly applied and do not cause crosshatching of the wound. Crosshatching occurs when it is necessary to pull skin together fairly snugly to approximate the edges. Sutures cut into the skin and cause scarring. Metal staples approximate the skin edges by applying pressure on either side of the wound and arching over the intervening skin. The metal does not touch the skin and cannot cause crosshatching.

NEEDLES

If the choice of suture is confusing, the choice of needles is totally chaotic. All needles are made of steel, although the inertness prized in steel sutures is sacrificed for hardness and ease of sharpening. However, unlike sutures, there are no universal standards for needle size and shape. Manufacturers are free to design and designate their own needles. There are hundreds of needles available, yet even a trained surgeon will be familiar with only a few dozen.

For the sake of order, all needles can be described in terms of four characteristics: eye, shape, point and cross section, and size (see box; also Fig. 3-1). Although there are no hard and fast rules governing needle selection, there are good reasons, in terms of these attributes, for selecting one needle over another.

Initially, all needles had eyes. Surgical needles, like surgical sutures, were originally borrowed from the tailoring trade. Ordinary milliner's needles, 4 and 5 cm in length, are sometimes still used. Eyed needles are versatile because they can be used with a great variety of sutures. Also they are less expensive, since one or two needles will serve for an entire row of sutures, and they can

NEEDLES

EYE

Eyed needle
Swaged needle
Loosely swaged (quick-release; "popoff")

SHAPE

Straight
3/8 circle
1/2 circle
5/8 circle

POINT AND CROSS SECTION

Taper needles
Cutting
Reverse cutting
Ground point wire needles (Ethicon Tapercut, Deknatel "K" needle)

SIZE: CURVED NEEDLES—MEASURED IN STRAIGHT LINE FROM HUB TO TIP

6 to 9 mm	Microsurgery, ophthalmology
1 to 1.5 cm	Cardiovascular surgery, pediatrics, urology, neurosurgery, dermatology
1.5 to 2.5 cm	Gastrointestinal, cardiovasular, general closure, soft tissue
2.5 to 4 cm	Heavy fascial closure, sternotomy closure
5 to 7 cm	Retension sutures

SIZE: STRAIGHT NEEDLES

4 to 6 cm (tapered)	Gastrointestinal, dermatology
4 to 6 cm (cutting)	Dermatology

Fig. 3-1. Parts of a needle.

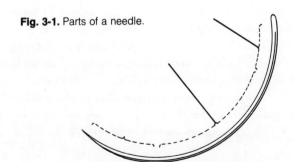

be cleaned and reused. Eyed needles are available in either straight or curved shapes and with either tapered or cutting points. The familiar Mayo needle is a fairly stout, tapered needle, available in several sizes in the 1.5 to 2.5 cm range, and is commonly used for suturing fascia. The Keith needle is a 6- to 7-cm straight-cutting needle used on the skin. But eyed needles also have a disadvantage. Since the eye of the needle needs to be somewhat larger than the suture, the needle is three or four times as thick as the suture. The needle makes a hole in the tissue that is larger than the suture. For skin and fascia, this is not a great disadvantage. It is unacceptable, however, for bowel, blood vessels, and other critical tissues. Swaged needles are used much more commonly.

The swaged needle is fastened to the end of the suture during manufacture and needs to be only slightly larger than the suture itself (Fig. 3-2). Since the needle is used for one length only of suture, it never becomes dull. For the same reason, it is expensive; for example, sutures with swaged needles for cardiovascular work may cost three or four dollars each.

In certain procedures, such as intestinal suturing, it is desirable to remove the needle from the suture quickly and easily. The swaged needle may be attached to the end of the suture loosely, so that a sharp tug will remove the needle after the suture has been placed through the tissue. These are called *controlled release* or *popoff* sutures.

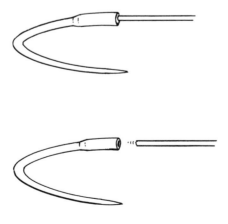

Fig. 3-2. Swaged needles.

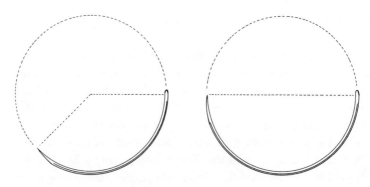

Fig. 3-3. Shapes of needles.

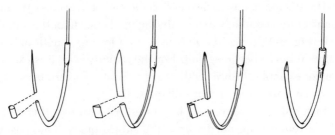

Fig. 3-4. Point and cross sections.

The shape of the needle (Fig. 3-3) is determined by how it is to be used. Straight needles are placed through the tissue by hand, while curved needles are placed with a needle holder. The 1/2 circle needle is most commonly used. Very fine needles, such as those used in vascular or ophthalmologic surgery, are usually 3/8 circle. Very large needles, such as the 6 to 7 cm curved needles used for placing retention sutures, are also 3/8 circle. Skin needles are usually 3/8 circle.

The point and cross section of the needle are determined by the type of tissue through which the needle is designed to pass (Fig. 3-4). For soft tissues and fascia, the tapered needle, round in cross section, is best. Using a cutting needle would produce small cuts along the suture tract, thus enlarging the holes. But for skin, which is very tough, cutting needles are much easier to use. The conventional cutting needle puts a small cut in the direction of pull of the suture; for this reason, reverse cutting needles, which have a flat edge in the direction of pull, are used in the skin. Cutting needles can be either curved or straight.

For sewing prosthetic grafts in the cardiovascular system, it is necessary to have a needle that is sharp enough to penetrate the tough graft but not damage the blood vessels. For this purpose the ground point wire needle has been developed. The saber point has sharp edges, but the body of the needle is round in cross section. The needle will pass through tissue without causing small cuts along the suture tract, but it will easily cut through graft material.

Finally, size is an obviously important characteristic of a needle. For the approximate sizes of needles used for different purposes see box on p. 34. The size is measured across the needle rather than along its curve; for example, a 1/2 circle and a 3/8 circle needle might seem to be the same size if measured from hub to point, despite the fact that the 1/2 circle needle would actually be 25% longer if measured along the needle.

KNOT TYING

The world is impressed by peculiar things. The most important technical expertise of the surgeon, for example, is knowing *how, where, when,* and most important, *why* to place sutures. However, to the layman, the most impressive characteristic is often the speed with which the surgeon ties knots. Actually, knot tying is a relatively simple and easily acquired skill that does not require great dexterity but simply adequate instruction and a moderate amount of practice. Instructions in knot tying are given in this section, but practice is up to the reader.

The dominant knot in surgery is the square knot. A properly tied square knot has 80% to 90% of the tensile strength of the uninterrupted strand; the square knot is the strongest knot for joining two strands of rope, string, or suture. In the illustration of the square knot (Fig. 3-5, *A*) it is evident that the two halves of the knot are mirror images. For that reason, the set of motions required to tie the first half will not do for the second half. Since the two hands are mirror images, the surgeon could use the same motion and alternate hands. However, most people find it more comfortable to tie consistently with one hand or the other.

The question of which hand to tie with always puzzles the beginner. Most people find it slightly easier to tie knots with the nondominant hand, so that right-handed persons usually tie with their left hands. For this reason, the drawings in this chapter are drawn to show the left hand tying the knots. To reverse the drawings, prop the book in front of a mirror.

Four methods of knot tying are described in the following pages. The first method is the so-called two-handed tie. This is actually a misnomer; most of the tying is still done with one hand, but the other hand is needed to manipulate the free end of the suture. The two-handed technique provides somewhat more control over the knot, is easier to tie under tension, and is easier to learn than the one-handed ties. In the illustrations, notice that the two-handed tie involves a great deal of wrist and forearm motion by the tying hand.

The second and third methods are one-handed techniques. These are slightly more difficult but are faster once learned. They are harder to tie under tension and not as easy to control. The one-handed techniques require more manual dexterity, because they call for independent action on the part of the long and ring fingers of the tying hand. The one-handed ties are accomplished with the fingers and with very little wrist motion. Most surgeons use only one or the other of the one-handed techniques. The techniques only differ in half of the knot; the first half of technique III is actually the second half of technique II.

Finally, the instrument tie is often used on the skin. It is especially useful for tying interrupted sutures with nylon or polyproplyene and is the common way of tying knots when sewing up skin lacerations. In practice, five or six throws are tied because polypropylene does not hold knots well. The instrument tie conserves suture, allowing one piece of suture with a swaged needle to be used six or eight times. Since it is difficult to hold tension while tying with this instrument, the surgeon's knot is especially useful, as shown in Fig. 3-5, *B*.

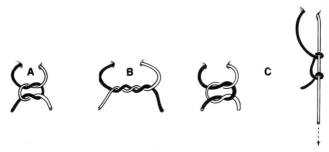

Fig. 3-5. Types of knots. **A,** Standard square knot. **B,** First half of surgeon's knot. **C,** Granny knot is really two half-hitches, as can be shown by pulling on one end before the knot is fully tightened. This results in one straight cord with two half-hitches tied around it. This is quite useful when a complete knot is to be tightened. On the other hand, its holding qualities are quite poor and it will slip if used by itself.

When surgeons speak of using "three knots" or "six knots" to tie a given suture, they mean the number of individual throws, or half-knots, not the number of completed square knots. Thus a complete square knot is called two knots. In tying a series of throws, it is best to alternate the throws in such a way as to tie complete square knots.

Two nonsquare knots are often used. The first is the surgeon's knot (Fig. 3-5, *B*). In this knot the first throw is doubled; that is, in the two-handed tie the manipulation of the first throw is repeated before tying down. This forms a first throw that will hold under moderate tension and is useful in tying skin and fascial sutures. The second throw is conventional.

The second knot is the two half hitches (Fig. 3-5, *C*). This is also called the granny knot, and is formed by tying two throws with the same hand motions. The granny knot is inferior to the square knot because it tends to slip. However, it allows the surgeon to tighten down a completed knot, as when tying skin sutures in the scalp. When this knot is used, a complete square knot should be tied on top of the granny knot.

Technique I: two-handed knot

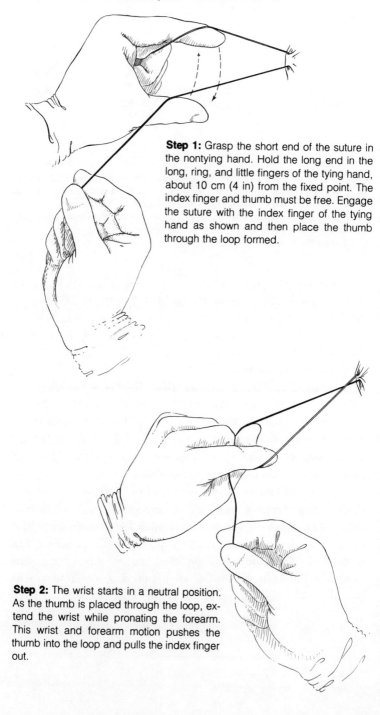

Step 1: Grasp the short end of the suture in the nontying hand. Hold the long end in the long, ring, and little fingers of the tying hand, about 10 cm (4 in) from the fixed point. The index finger and thumb must be free. Engage the suture with the index finger of the tying hand as shown and then place the thumb through the loop formed.

Step 2: The wrist starts in a neutral position. As the thumb is placed through the loop, extend the wrist while pronating the forearm. This wrist and forearm motion pushes the thumb into the loop and pulls the index finger out.

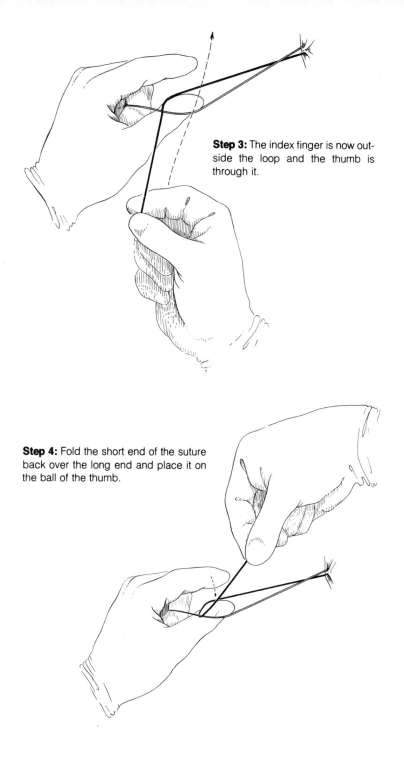

Step 3: The index finger is now outside the loop and the thumb is through it.

Step 4: Fold the short end of the suture back over the long end and place it on the ball of the thumb.

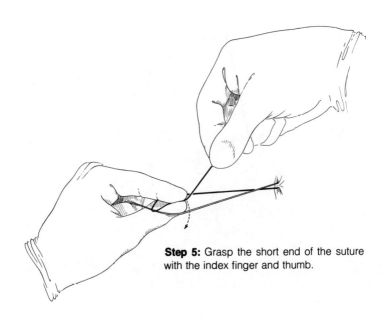

Step 5: Grasp the short end of the suture with the index finger and thumb.

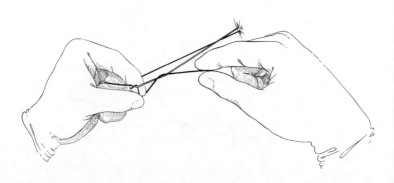

Step 6: Flex the wrist.

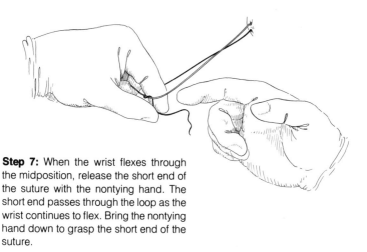

Step 7: When the wrist flexes through the midposition, release the short end of the suture with the nontying hand. The short end passes through the loop as the wrist continues to flex. Bring the nontying hand down to grasp the short end of the suture.

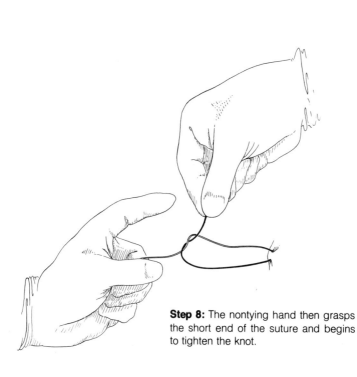

Step 8: The nontying hand then grasps the short end of the suture and begins to tighten the knot.

Step 9: Use the index finger of the tying hand to push the knot down to the fixed point and tighten it. This avoids tension on the fixed point, which may be a relatively fragile vessel, or on some other structure that might be damaged by excessive tension. Tighten the knot flat as shown, even if it is necessary to cross the hands to do so; if the first throw is not placed flat, the completed knot may slip.

Step 10: Begin the second half of the technique from the final position reached after tightening the first half and without changing either hand's grasp on the suture. Engage the suture with the thumb of the tying hand.

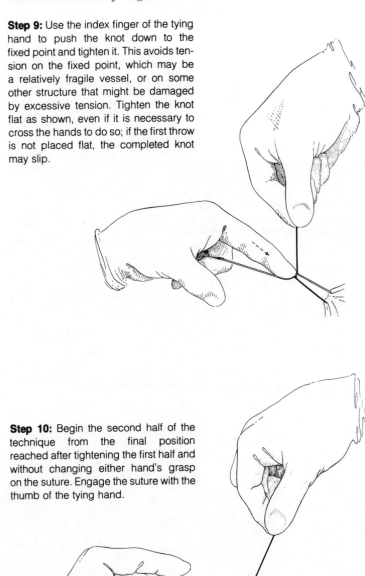

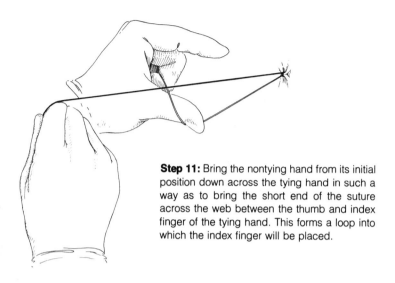

Step 11: Bring the nontying hand from its initial position down across the tying hand in such a way as to bring the short end of the suture across the web between the thumb and index finger of the tying hand. This forms a loop into which the index finger will be placed.

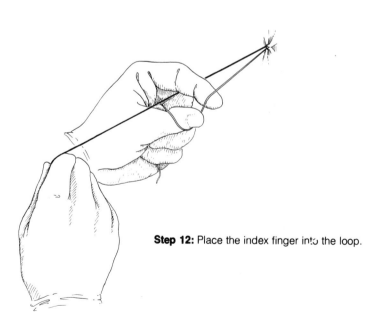

Step 12: Place the index finger into the loop.

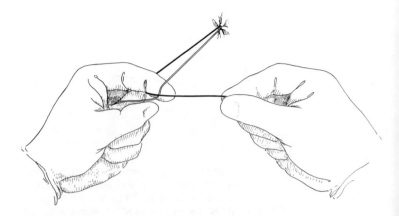

Step 13: Flex the wrist. This pushes the index finger further into the loop while withdrawing the thumb. Then move the nontying hand back toward its original position, folding the short end of the suture along the ball of the index finger.

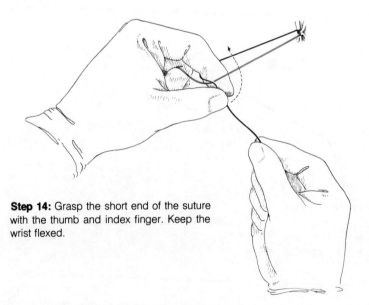

Step 14: Grasp the short end of the suture with the thumb and index finger. Keep the wrist flexed.

Step 15: Release the short end of the suture and extend the wrist. This brings the short end through the loop. Move the nontying hand up.

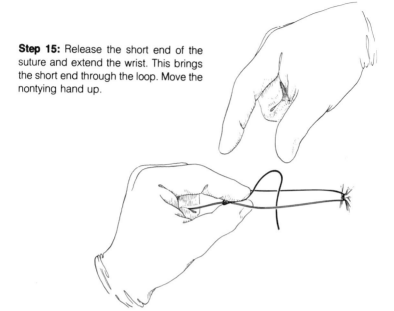

Step 16: Grasp the short end of the suture as it is released by the thumb and index finger of the tying hand.

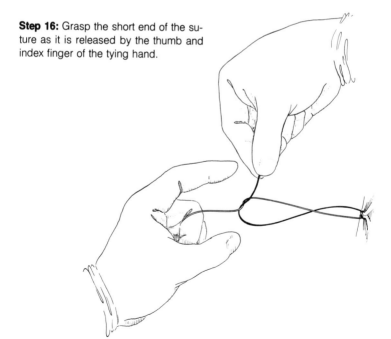

Step 17: Push the knot down with the index finger of the tying hand.

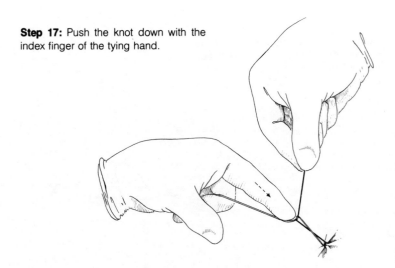

Technique II: one-handed tie

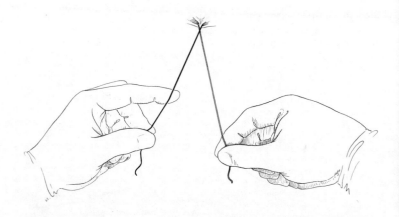

Step 1: In contrast to the two-handed tie, grasp the short end of the suture with the long finger of the tying hand and the long end with the nontying hand. Pass the index finger of the tying hand under the short end of the suture. The palm of the tying hand faces down. Notice that the suture is crossed at the fixed point.

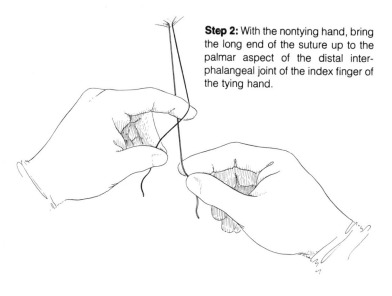

Step 2: With the nontying hand, bring the long end of the suture up to the palmar aspect of the distal interphalangeal joint of the index finger of the tying hand.

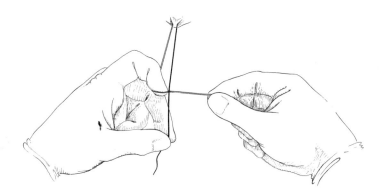

Step 3: Without otherwise moving the hands, strongly flex the index finger of the tying hand. In doing this, it is important to keep the thumb and long finger, which are grasping the short end of the suture firmly extended.

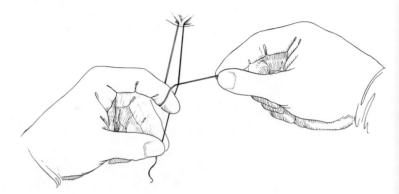

Step 4: Move the index finger up and over the short end of the suture, which should still be held fixed by the thumb and long finger.

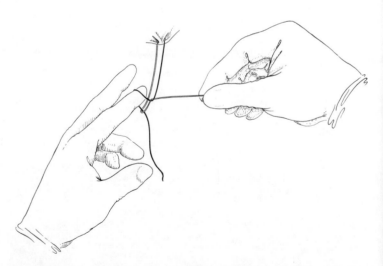

Step 5: With the index finger, pull the short end of the suture through the loop formed by the long end, while the thumb and long finger release the short end. The long finger moves up next to the index finger, where it will secure the short end.

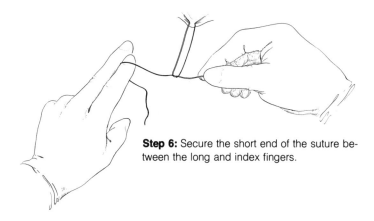

Step 6: Secure the short end of the suture between the long and index fingers.

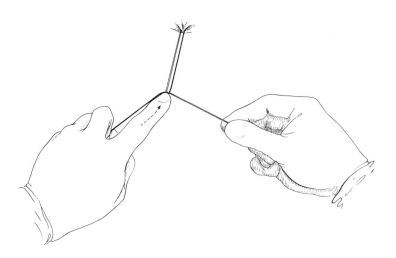

Step 7: Bring the thumb over to the long finger to grasp the short end of the suture and push the knot down with the index finger.

Note: The second half of Technique II is the same as the first half of Technique III (through Step 7).

Technique III: one-handed tie

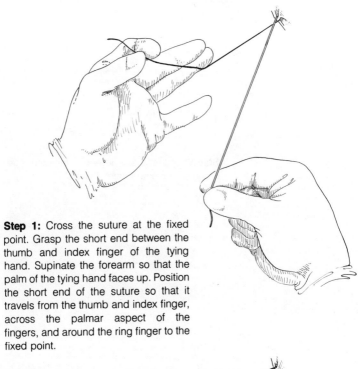

Step 1: Cross the suture at the fixed point. Grasp the short end between the thumb and index finger of the tying hand. Supinate the forearm so that the palm of the tying hand faces up. Position the short end of the suture so that it travels from the thumb and index finger, across the palmar aspect of the fingers, and around the ring finger to the fixed point.

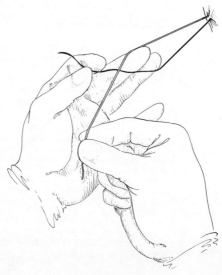

Step 2: Cross the nontying hand in front of the tying hand to position the end of the suture along the radial aspect of the long finger, crossing the short end of the suture at a point about halfway from the thumb to the ring finger.

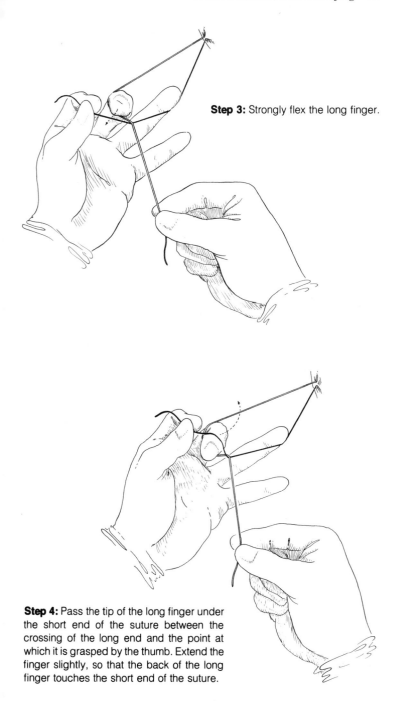

Step 3: Strongly flex the long finger.

Step 4: Pass the tip of the long finger under the short end of the suture between the crossing of the long end and the point at which it is grasped by the thumb. Extend the finger slightly, so that the back of the long finger touches the short end of the suture.

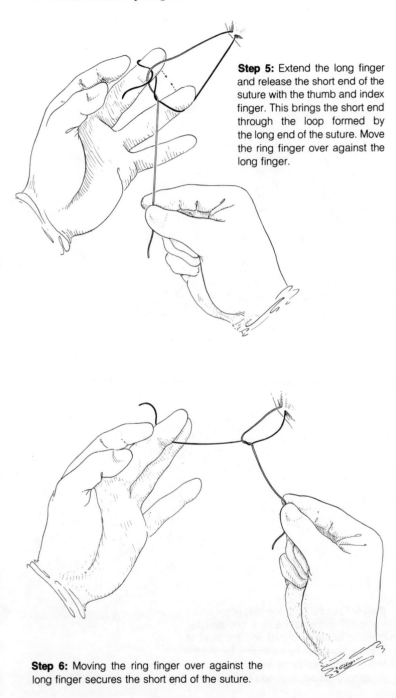

Step 5: Extend the long finger and release the short end of the suture with the thumb and index finger. This brings the short end through the loop formed by the long end of the suture. Move the ring finger over against the long finger.

Step 6: Moving the ring finger over against the long finger secures the short end of the suture.

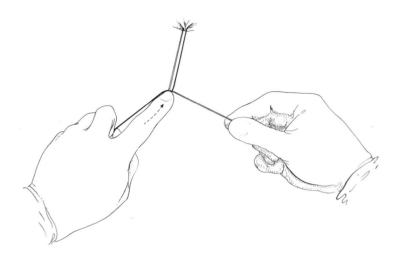

Step 7: Grasp the short end of the suture between the thumb and long fingers of the tying hand and push the knot down with the index finger.

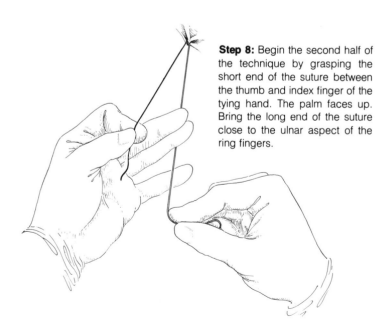

Step 8: Begin the second half of the technique by grasping the short end of the suture between the thumb and index finger of the tying hand. The palm faces up. Bring the long end of the suture close to the ulnar aspect of the ring fingers.

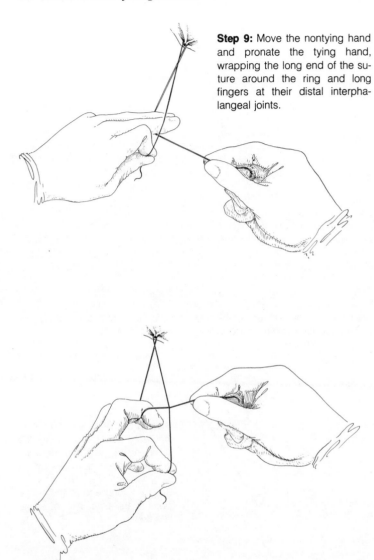

Step 9: Move the nontying hand and pronate the tying hand, wrapping the long end of the suture around the ring and long fingers at their distal interphalangeal joints.

Step 10: Strongly flex the ring and long fingers. Keeping the thumb firmly extended, pronate the hand somewhat (not fully). The ring and long fingers pull the long end of the suture away from the point at which it crosses the short end. Move the nontying hand slightly toward the tying hand to allow the ring and long fingers to pull the long end of the suture in toward the palm of the tying hand. Notice the position at which the short and long ends of the suture cross. It is well away from the tying hand. This is the most difficult part of the technique.

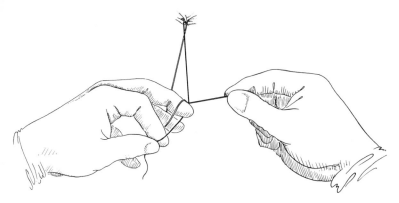

Step 11: Separate the ring and long fingers slightly and extend them somewhat. Grasp the short end of the suture between the point at which it crosses the long end and the point at which it is held by the thumb and index finger. This maneuver is relatively easy, if the previous step was done properly.

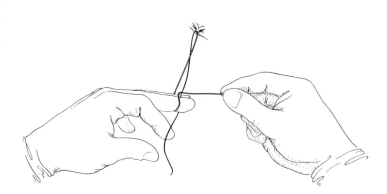

Step 12: While holding the short end of the suture between the ring and long fingers, release it with the thumb and index fingers.

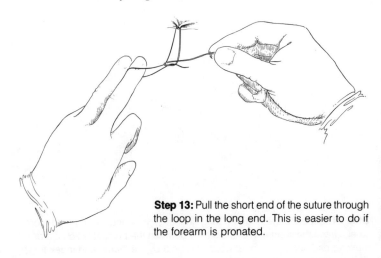

Step 13: Pull the short end of the suture through the loop in the long end. This is easier to do if the forearm is pronated.

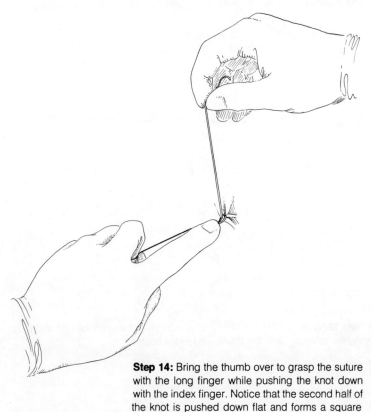

Step 14: Bring the thumb over to grasp the suture with the long finger while pushing the knot down with the index finger. Notice that the second half of the knot is pushed down flat and forms a square knot with the first half.

Technique IV: instrument tie (surgeon's knot)

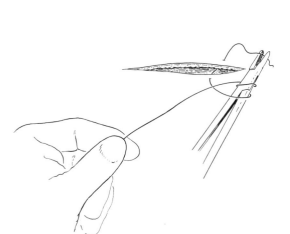

Step 1: Hold the end of the suture that has a swaged needle in the nontying hand. Pull the suture through the skin until about 2 cm of free end remains. Wrap the suture around the needle holder twice.

Step 2: Grasp the free end of the suture in the needle holder.

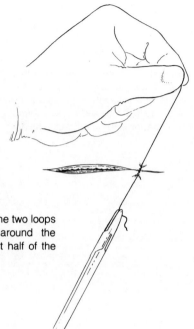

Step 3: Pull the free end through the two loops that were previously wrapped around the needle holder and tighten the first half of the surgeon's knot.

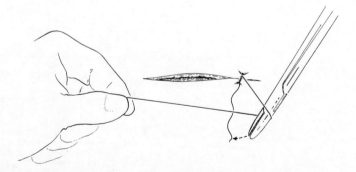

Step 4: Wrap the long end of the suture once around the needle holder in the opposite direction from Step 1. Grasp the short end in the jaws of the needle holder.

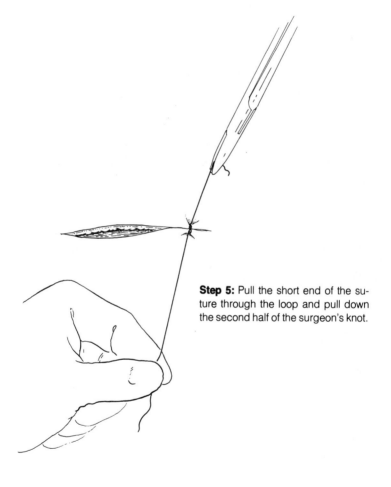

Step 5: Pull the short end of the suture through the loop and pull down the second half of the surgeon's knot.

4

Anesthesia

Most of the procedures outlined in this book can be performed under local anesthesia. Local anesthetic agents are effective in alleviating the pain of surgery; patients, however, are usually still aware that a surgical procedure is being performed. Stereotactic and pressure senses, though dulled, tend to persist. The practitioner should remember that even the most minor procedures produce substantial anxiety on the part of the patient. A simple and clear explanation of the intended procedure with progress reports during the procedure can greatly allay these anxieties. Some patients, however, require a mild, short-acting sedative for even the most minor procedure. Diazepam (Valium) in 5 to 10 mg doses is an effective premedication that may be given intravenously if rapid onset is desired. Infants and small children usually require some form of preoperative medication.

ANESTHETIC AGENTS

Though numerous anesthetic agents are available, the practitioner should become familiar with two or three of the most useful drugs. For the types of procedures described in this book, procaine and lidocaine are the agents of choice. Bupivacaine is important because of its prolonged duration of action.

Procaine (Novocain)
  Duration—approximately 1 hour
  Maximum dose—700 mg
  Recommended concentration—0.5% infiltration and field
    block; 2% nerve block
Lidocaine (Xylocaine)
  Duration—approximately 3 hours
  Maximum dose—300 mg (7 mg/kg/body weight)
  Recommended concentration—0.5% infiltration and field
    block; 1% nerve block

Bupivacaine (Marcaine)
  Duration—approximately 8 hours
  Maximum dose—175 mg
  Recommended concentration—0.25% infiltration and field
    block; 0.5% nerve block

All of the above agents have a rapid onset, which occurs in 3 to 10 minutes. In addition, most agents are available with a vasoconstrictor, typically epinephrine in a fixed concentration. The addition of the vasoconstrictor decreases the rate of absorption, thereby lessening toxicity and allowing the practitioner to give a higher total dose of the anesthetic agent. Vasoconstrictors also prolong the duration of anesthesia (about 50%) and decrease the amount of bleeding from the operative site.

When using infiltration anesthesia with vasoconstrictors, one should be extremely careful to ensure adequate surgical hemostasis, because as these agents wear off, bleeding can occur and complicate an otherwise perfect procedure. Vasoconstrictors are *absolutely contraindicated* for blocks or infiltration in peripheral appendages such as the fingers, toes, or ears, where they can cause ischemic necrosis. They should be avoided in patients with hypertensive, cardiac, and peripheral vascular disease.

Complications

Local anesthetics are potent pharmacologic agents and should be used only when resuscitative drugs and equipment are immediately available. The safety and effectiveness of local anesthetics depend on:

1. Correct dosage: use the smallest amount of agent necessary to obtain the desired level of anesthesia
2. Correct technique: slow injection with frequent aspiration
3. Proper precautions: immediate availability of emergency medication and resuscitation equipment
4. Alertness for reactions and complications

The most common complication associated with local anesthetics is overdosage. This should be avoided by careful attention to the amount and concentration of agent and the technique of administration. Overdosage often follows accidental injection into a vein.

The initial signs of overdosage are:
1. Irregular pulse
2. Either rapid or slowed pulse
3. Hypotension
4. Shallow, rapid respirations

The initial symptoms of overdosage are:
1. Excitement and apprehension (may be very transient)
2. Headache
3. Nausea and vomiting
4. Muscle twitching

These early signs and symptoms can rapidly progress to convulsions, unconsciousness, respiratory depression, and circulatory failure. At the first signs of overdosage, the practitioner must stop administration of the agent and start oxygen by mask. Maintenance of an adequate airway with immediate endotracheal intubation, if necessary, may be lifesaving.

Hypotension often requires cardiovascular support with phenylephrine (Neo-Synephrine), 1 to 2 mg in 10 ml saline given intravenously. For persistent hypotension, 20 mg of phenylephrine in 500 ml of 5% dextrose in water, given intravenously, is usually effective in maintaining blood pressure. Convulsions usually respond to improved oxygenation. If they persist, however, diazepam, given intravenously in 5 mg doses, will eventually control the seizures.

Sensitivity reactions are occasionally seen. They are marked by typical allergic responses, such as hives, itching, wheezing, hypotension, and angioneurotic edema. If these symptoms occur, stop the administration of the anesthetic immediately. Itching, hives, and edema usually respond to 25 to 50 mg of diphenhydramine (Benadryl) intravenously. Sensitivity reactions are life-threatening if the edema involves the larynx. Danger signs are itching of the throat, increasing hoarseness, and inspiratory stridor. In addition to diphenhydramine, epinephrine (0.3 to 0.5 ml of 1:1000) should be given subcutaneously and repeated in 15 minutes if necessary. Mild, isolated wheezing, typical of asthma, will usually respond to aminophylline (250 to 500 mg) administered by a slow intravenous infusion.

Anaphylactic shock is remarkably uncommon, but when it does occur it represents a life-threatening emergency. Immediately give 0.5 to 1 ml of 1:1000 epinephrine subcutaneously and call for assistance. Place an intravenous line, and give 0.1 mg of epinephrine (0.1 ml of 1:1000) slowly. If hypotension persists, add 300 mg of metaraminol bitartrate (Aramine) to the intravenous solution. Titrate the rate of administration to the blood pressure response.

Maintain an adequate airway. Start artificial respiration until oxygen can be delivered with positive pressure through a mask. Be prepared to intubate the patient.

All patients who become hypotensive should be admitted to the hospital for further care and observation. Patients with minor reactions can be discharged under a physician's care and should be given oral antihistamines for several days.

ANESTHETIC TECHNIQUES

The minor surgical procedures described in this book require facility with a few anesthetic techniques. As important as the anesthetic agent itself are the few minutes the good practitioner will spend with the patient describing the technique, keeping the patient informed of progress, and essentially talking the patient through the procedure.

Infiltration anesthesia is the most useful and widely used technique for minor surgery. The surgeon first raises an intradermal wheal with a small amount of anesthetic through a 25- to 30-gauge needle. The anesthetic is then injected through the wheal into the subcutaneous tissue surrounding the proposed operative site. Depending on the area to be infiltrated, the same needle or a longer (2- to 3-inch) 22-gauge needle is used. Larger areas often require more than one skin wheal (Fig. 4-1). When agents are injected into the subcutaneous tissue, frequent aspiration will prevent injection directly into vessels. In lacerations, direct absorption can be avoided by infiltrating the perimeter.

Field block is another useful technique. It provides "a field of anesthesia" around the proposed operative site. It is especially recommended when large areas need to be anesthetized or when adjacent areas would require separate infiltration. After prepar-

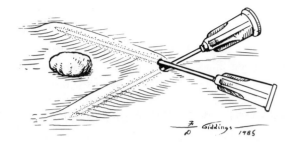

Fig. 4-1. Technique of raising anesthetic skin wheals in preparation for infiltration.

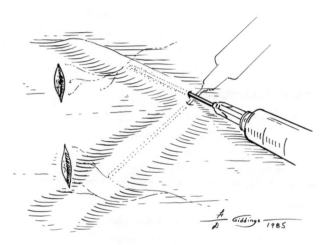

Fig. 4-2. Technique of field block.

ing the operative site, raise a skin wheal with a dilute anesthetic agent (0.5% to 1% lidocaine) along the perimeter of the proposed field. Insert a long 22-gauge needle through this wheal. Direct it along the proposed perimeter, just subdermally, injecting anesthetic while advancing the needle. Never insert the needle to its hub, since this is its weakest point, and if it breaks the needle would be buried in the tissues. To continue the perimeter injection, partially withdraw the needle and redirect it as in Fig. 4-2. By using this technique, a large area can be blocked through one wheal. If additional perimeter requires infiltration, insert the needle through an area that has already been anesthetized. After

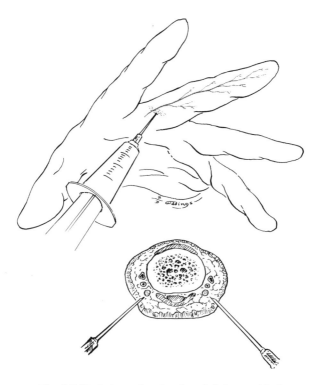

Fig. 4-3. Technique of performing digital nerve block.

infiltrating the perimeter, inject the deeper tissues along this perimeter line down to the fascia.

Some procedures, because of their specific location, lend themselves to the use of nerve or regional blocks. This technique calls for the blocking of a specific somatic nerve, providing anesthesia over the distal distribution of the nerve.

A particularly useful block is the digital block (Fig. 4-3), which provides complete anesthesia of a finger or toe. The digital nerves lie close to the bone toward the volar side. After preparing the skin, usually of the entire hand, raise bilateral skin wheals on the lateral aspects of the finger just distal to the metacarpophalangeal joint. Insert the needle toward the general position of the nerve and inject a small amount of anesthetic agent. Then infiltrate smaller amounts of anesthetic in a fanlike pattern from this point. Never use an agent with an added vasoconstrictor for a

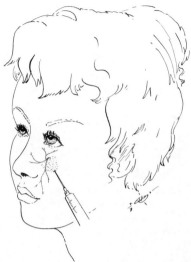

Fig. 4-4. Technique of blocking infraorbital nerve.

Fig. 4-5. Technique of blocking mental nerve.

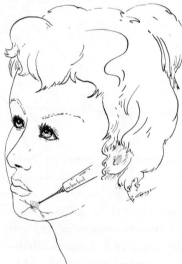

digital block, because severe ischemia and even gangrene might result. A small rubber band tourniquet helps to produce a bloodless field that makes precise technical procedures possible. Never leave the tourniquet on for longer than 30 to 40 minutes.

Another useful block, the infraorbital block, provides excellent anesthesia to the malar area (Fig. 4-4). After suitable preoperative preparation of the site, palpate the infraorbital ridge ap-

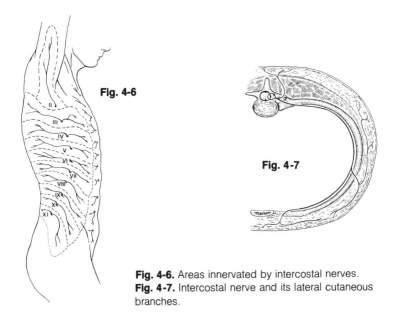

Fig. 4-6

Fig. 4-7

Fig. 4-6. Areas innervated by intercostal nerves.
Fig. 4-7. Intercostal nerve and its lateral cutaneous branches.

proximately 1 inch from the facial midline. Make an anesthetic skin wheal approximately 1 cm below this point and direct the needle toward the foramen, injecting about 2 ml of anesthetic as it is advanced. When the foramen is encountered, the patient will experience paresthesia along the distribution of the nerve. Once the foramen is entered, inject another 0.5 ml of the anesthetic. For procedures on the lower jaw or lower lip, a mental block is often useful. The mental foramen is located about 1 inch from the midline in the midportion of the mandible (Fig. 4-5). Insert the needle superiorly and lateral to the foramen and inject anesthetic solution as the needle is advanced toward the foramen. When paresthesia signifies that the nerve has been encountered, inject an additional 1 ml of anesthetic. Next advance the needle a short distance into the foramen, injecting another 0.5 ml.

The intercostal block provides excellent anesthesia for minor procedures on the lower chest and upper abdomen (Fig. 4-6) and affords temporary pain relief following rib fracture. For the most effective anesthesia, inject the nerve before the origin of the lateral cutaneous branches (Fig. 4-7). This requires injecting the

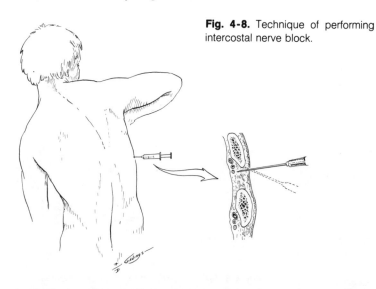

Fig. 4-8. Technique of performing intercostal nerve block.

intercostal nerves at the posterior angle of the rib, about halfway between the posterior axillary line and the spine. The scapula blocks access to spaces above the seventh intercostal space. For these areas, block the nerve in the posterior axillary line. Adequate anesthesia can often be obtained by blocks in the posterior axillary line with less risk of complication. The landmarks are more obvious and the needle path is shorter.

Minor procedures on the thoracic wall or relief of pain in fractures usually requires anesthetic block of one or two intercostal nerves both above and below the involved dermatome. The intercostal nerves lie deep to the midplane of the rib close to its inferior margin (Fig. 4-8) and exceedingly close to the pleural cavity. To block the nerves, raise the typical skin wheal and direct the 22-gauge needle toward the inferior portion of the rib. When contact is made with the rib, withdraw the needle a short distance and direct it more inferiorly so that it just slips under the inferior margin of the rib. Advance the needle no more than one eighth of an inch past the inferior margin of the rib. At this point aspirate to make sure the needle has not entered the lung (return of air) or an intercostal vessel. If there is no return on aspiration, inject 3 to 5 ml of anesthetic solution. Bupivacaine will provide long-lasting analgesia for fractured ribs.

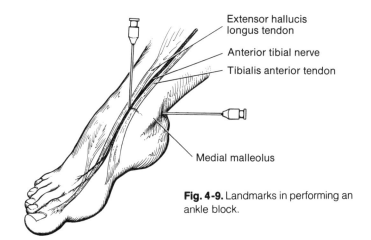

Extensor hallucis
longus tendon

Anterior tibial nerve

Tibialis anterior tendon

Medial malleolus

Fig. 4-9. Landmarks in performing an ankle block.

An ankle block provides excellent anesthesia for procedures on the foot. The anterior and posterior tibial nerves are blocked at the level of the malleoli. To block the tibial nerve, insert a needle to the bone between the anterior tibialis and the extensor hallucis longis, withdraw slightly, and inject 2 to 5 ml of anesthetic agent. Block the posterior nerve similarly, inserting the needle to the bone on the medial side of the ankle just medial to the calcaneus tendon, withdrawing slightly, and injecting 2 to 5 ml of anesthetic agent (Fig. 4-9).

Infiltrate the posterolateral compartment with 5 ml, to block fibers of the sural nerve. Complete the block with a circumferential subcutaneous infiltration again at the level of the malleoli.

Bier block

For procedures on the forearm or hand, the Bier block, or regional intravenous block, has become popular. This block requires two pneumatic tourniquets placed on the upper arm. Insert an intravenous cannula distally and exsanguinate the arm with an Esmarch bandage. Inflate the proximal tourniquet to a level 100 torr above the systolic pressure. Inject lidocaine (3 mg/kg) or bupivacaine (1.5 mg/kg) through the intravenous cannula. The distal tourniquet now lies on an anesthetized field. If pain develops at the site of the proximal tourniquet, inflate the distal tourniquet and then release the proximal tourniquet.

This block provides excellent anesthesia plus a bloodless operative field but has three drawbacks:

1. Because of "tourniquet time," procedure should be completed within 1 hour.
2. Once blood flow is reestablished, anesthesia is rapidly lost. The procedure must either be totally completed in a bloodless field (with the possibility of bleeding into the wound) or completed with a supplemental local anesthesia.
3. The tourniquet must remain inflated for at least 25 minutes to allow for full binding of the agent. Tourniquet failure at an early stage can result in washout and severe toxicity.

For the above reasons the intravenous block is best performed and monitored by an anesthesiologist.

• • •

These blocks represent only a few of the many available. They are probably the most useful and frequently used regional blocks, and the practitioner should become proficient with these simpler blocks before attempting the more sophisticated ones.

5

Care of the acute wound

The minor acute wound is one of the most frequent problems confronting the practitioner. Fortunately most of the injuries are easily handled by following a few basic principles of management.

EVALUATION OF THE WOUND

History—Important in determining type of wound care needed

How: Aids in assessment of possible contamination by retained foreign bodies

Where: Further elucidates the possibility of contamination

When: Information useful in deciding to close the wound primarily or to leave it open

Examination—

1. Location: Important as an indication of the possibility of injury to deeper structures and must be considered in planning for wound closure. In general, connective tissue bundles tend to follow a predictable course within the dermis (Fig. 5-1). Wound closures running parallel to these lines tend to remain thin, and wounds across these tension lines tend to expand.

2. Exploration: Gentle exploration must be performed to rule out injury to deeper structures and to locate retained foreign material and devitalized tissue.

3. An x-ray examination should be done if there is a possibility of retained material.

PRINCIPLES OF WOUND CARE
Debridement

The first and most important principle of wound care, and unfortunately the one most frequently overlooked, is adequate

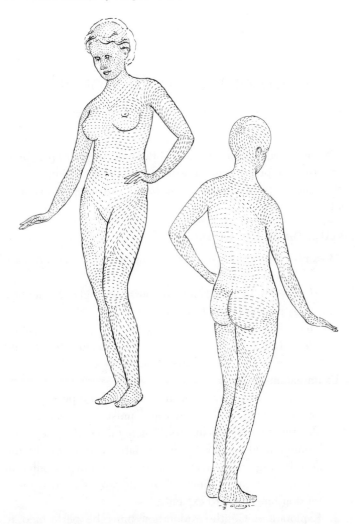

Fig. 5-1. Langer's lines—the general course of the bundles of connective tissue within the dermis. Wounds that cross these lines tend to be widened by the inherent tension.

and thorough debridement. Devitalized tissue and retained foreign material act as focal points for infection and can ruin otherwise precise and meticulous care. Jagged edges must be removed by sharp dissection before closure is attempted (Fig. 5-2). Copious irrigation with normal saline is extremely helpful in flushing out retained foreign material and devitalized tissue.

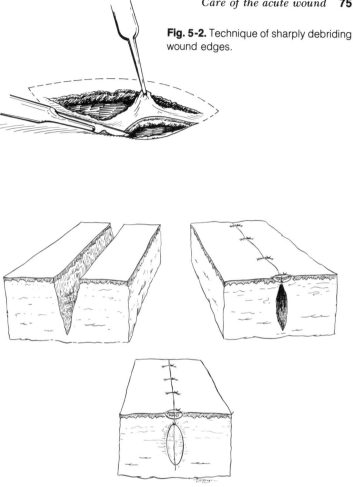

Fig. 5-2. Technique of sharply debriding wound edges.

Fig. 5-3. Technique for eliminating dead space by using a deep suture.

Closure

Given a clean incised wound, primary closure is indicated if the wound is less than 8 hours old. This form of closure entails the approximation of the wound edges with either tape or sutures. (Tape closure is effective only in very superficial wounds.) For deeper wounds or in widely separated wounds, the subcutaneous layers must be closed to eliminate dead space and relieve tension on the skin closure (Fig. 5-3). In using sutures for primary closure, the following principles should be kept in mind:

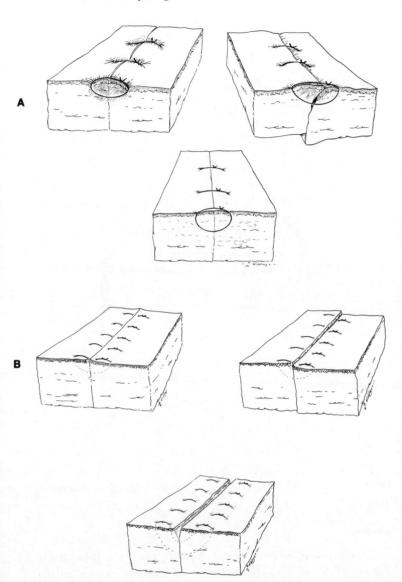

Fig. 5-4. Effects of suture tension.

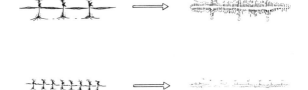

Fig. 5-5. The effects of suture size and placement.

1. Sutures are meant only to approximate the skin edges. If they are tied too tightly, ischemia or overlapping wound edges will result (Fig. 5-4). (Approximate—do not strangulate.) Remember that some edema will occur following closure and a precisely approximated wound might become too tight.
2. Use the smallest size suture necessary to maintain closure. This is especially important in exposed areas where cosmetic considerations are important.
3. Small sutures placed close together accomplish the same purpose as large sutures placed farther apart and create a more cosmetic closure with less scarring (Fig. 5-5).
4. Tension is best handled by using subcutaneous absorbable sutures.

The most useful and commonly used suture technique is the simple over-and-over suture. This can be used as an interrupted suture (Fig. 5-6) or as a continuous suture (Fig. 5-7). The difficulty with the continuous suture is that if the strand breaks the entire wound may separate. In suturing, forceps should be used as infrequently as possible to avoid further trauma to the wound. The needle should enter and exit the skin at right angles, and the natural curve of the needle should be followed. The final knot that completes the continuous suture is shown in Fig. 5-8.

Precise edge approximation is more easily obtained with the vertical mattress stitch (Figs. 5-4, *B*, and 5-9). The near bites are placed close to the wound edges (1 mm) and provide for precise approximation, although, the bites farther away (7 mm) relieve

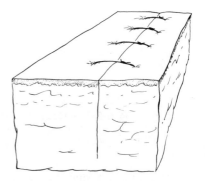

Fig. 5-6. Simple interrupted sutures.

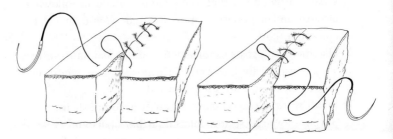

Fig. 5-7. Examples of continuous or "running" sutures.

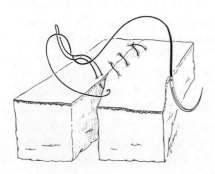

Fig. 5-8. Technique for tying off the continuous suture.

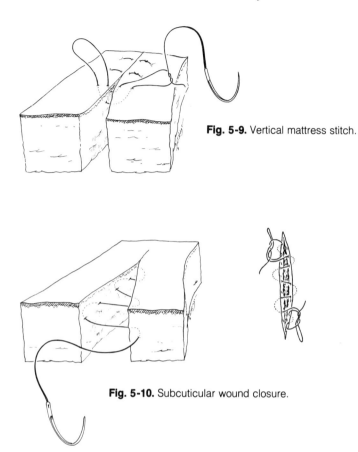

Fig. 5-9. Vertical mattress stitch.

Fig. 5-10. Subcuticular wound closure.

the tension. This type of closure is extremely useful on the trunk and abdomen, and with large wounds.

As more facility with wound closure technique is developed, the subcuticular closure should be tried (Fig. 5-10). This is an excellent cosmetic closure because it eliminates the crosshatching caused by suture marks. As shown in Fig. 5-10, it is entirely buried, including the knot, so that an absorbable type of suture is used, such as 4-0 or 5-0 Dexon or Vicryl. The wound is then reinforced with "Steri-strips" applied to the skin.

Suture removal, when performed properly, should be a virtually painless procedure. First swab the wound with alcohol or

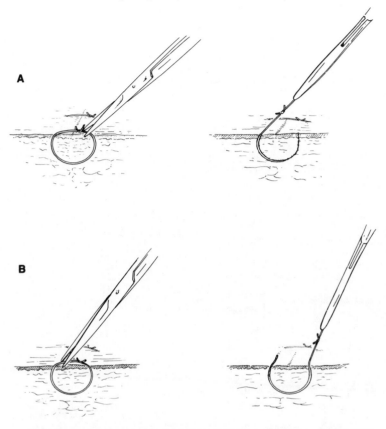

Fig. 5-11. Technique of suture removal. **A,** Proper technique. **B,** Improper technique illustrating source of contamination.

an antiseptic and gently remove the dried exudate. Grasp the knot or the loose ends of the sutures with a thumb forceps and gently elevate. Cut the suture with a scissors or a No. 11 scalpel blade where it enters the skin (Fig. 5-11, *A*). This eliminates pulling contaminated sutures through the suture tract (Fig. 5-11, *B*).

Types and management

Any type of wound with a small entrance and a deep tract is best left open to drain, because these wounds may develop deep infections. It is often wise to excise the skin around the entrance of the wound and to insert a small gauze wick into the wound to

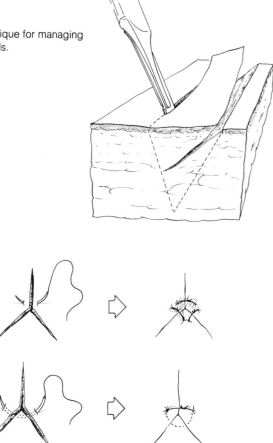

Fig. 5-12. Technique for managing tangential wounds.

Fig. 5-13. Technique for managing stellate using a **U** stitch to avoid ischemia of wound edges.

ensure drainage. Tangentially incised wounds are often difficult to close with precise approximation of skin edges. Excise the entire wound (Fig. 5-12) to obtain a good cosmetic closure. V-shaped fragments of tissue have a precarious blood supply and should either be excised or closed with a **U** stitch that preserves the blood supply to the apex (Fig. 5-13).

Many infected wounds require hospitalization and systemic antibiotics.

Location

Face. The excellent blood supply to the tissues of the face ensures prompt healing of clean wounds. However, because of the exposed nature of the wound, extra care has to be taken to ensure the best cosmetic results.

1. Debride only obviously necrotic tissue.
2. Obtain excellent hemostasis.
3. Do not shave the eyebrow.
4. Use natural facial borders for aid in aligning tissue (for example, the vermilion border of lip and the eyebrow). Be precise (Fig. 5-14).
5. If at all possible, try to design the closure so that the resulting wound will lie in the plane of the natural folds of the face. All scars contract, but scars placed parallel to the natural folds are less noticeable.
6. Use 5-0 or 6-0 monofilament suture placed no more than 2.5 mm apart and 2.5 mm from the wound edge.

Because the cosmetic results of unclosed wounds on the face are poor, and because the good facial blood supply affords an excellent chance for healing, many surgeons will primarily close facial wounds that are more than 8 hours old. Some will even close animal bites. Before a facial wound is left open to heal on its own, the advice of a general or plastic surgeon should be sought.

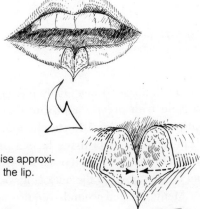

Fig. 5-14. Technique for the precise approximation of the vermillion border of the lip.

Wounds involving the eyelid, the lacrimal apparatus, the parotid duct, and branches of the facial nerves as well as extensive wounds require the services of a trained general or plastic surgeon.

Hands. Minor lacerations of the hands are extremely common and usually present no real problem. However, be aware that what looks like a minor laceration of the hand may indeed represent a major injury. Thoroughly and systematically evaluate all hand injuries under sterile conditions before any anesthetic is given. For even minor injuries, pay particular attention to any loss of either motor or sensory nerve function or evidence of tendon or vascular injury. The patient will often complain of areas of numbness, but the practitioner should check distally with a needle to definitively rule out nerve damage. Damage to the extensor tendon of the hand will render the patient unable to fully extend one or more fingers. Test the superficial flexor tendons by having the patient flex one finger at a time while the other fingers are held extended (Fig. 5-15). The deep flexor tendons are tested by having the patient flex the distal phalanx, while the remainder of the finger is held extended (Fig. 5-16). The presence of either real or suspected nerve/tendon injury necessitates the expert care of a trained surgeon.

Because of the contraction processes inherent in wound healing, wounds across flexor surfaces can lead to contracture and limitation of full extension. These wounds should be converted to transverse wounds to prevent this problem (Fig. 5-17).

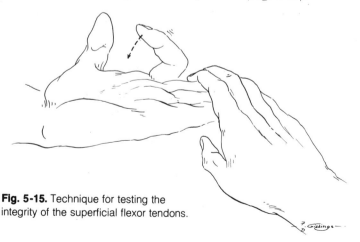

Fig. 5-15. Technique for testing the integrity of the superficial flexor tendons.

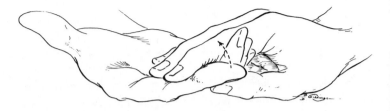

Fig. 5-16. Technique for testing the integrity of the deep flexor tendons.

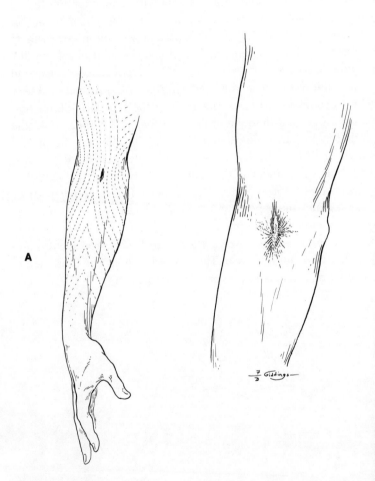

Fig. 5-17. Wounds across flexor surfaces. **A,** Results of wounds across flexor surface.

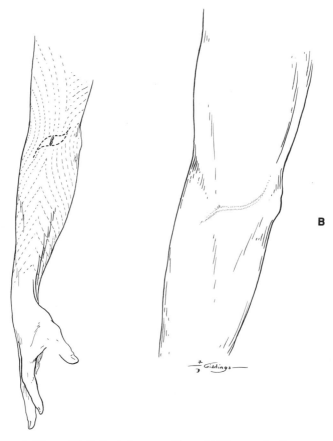

Fig. 5-17, cont'd. B, Technique used to avoid this complication.

DRESSINGS AND SPLINTS

In most instances the dressing applied to most minor primarily closed wounds should be minimal. It is used to prevent further contamination and to protect the area from further trauma. If the wound is small enough, a Band-Aid will usually suffice. For larger areas, use one or two gauze sponges held in place by tape. In the past, difficult areas to bandage required the practitioner to learn complex taping and bandaging techniques. This process is greatly simplified by the use of elastic netting. This material can be fashioned to secure a dressing to almost any portion of the body (Fig. 5-18).

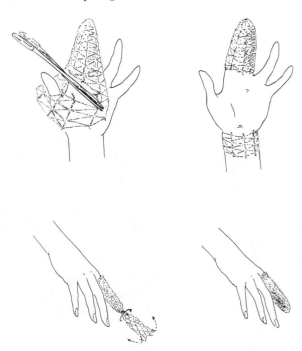

Fig. 5-18. Techniques for using elastic netting.

A small strip of a nonadherent plastic will prevent sutures and wound exudate from adhering to the gauze sponges. Avoid the use of bulky or impermeable dressings because they inhibit the circulation of air and the accumulation of perspiration and wound exudate under the dressing can macerate the skin and become infected. No antibiotic ointment is necessary.

Facial wounds in adults are often best treated without dressing. Have the patient cleanse the area daily with a little hydrogen peroxide to remove the exudate.

Dress small *scalp wounds* with a small amount of colloidion applied to the wound. This is a liquid that dries into a film, thus protecting the wound. Tape or other adhesive material used on the scalp often becomes entangled in the hair and is difficult to remove. Larger dressings of gauze can be held in place by a cap made from elastic netting.

Hand wounds pose a more difficult problem. Use Band-Aids for the minor wounds. For larger wounds, use an elastic net to

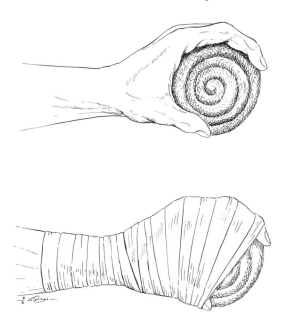

Fig. 5-19. "Position of function."

hold the dressing in place. This is most effective when only one finger has to be dressed; however, when there are multiple lacerations or when the wounds have to be treated surgically, it is best to include the entire hand in a dressing. Pad the entire hand and wrist with gauze between the fingers, then wrap with a loose gauze net such as Kerlix, leaving an extra amount of gauze in the palm. This maintains the hand in the so-called *position of function* (Fig. 5-19) with the fingers slightly flexed and the thumb in line with the radius. Secure this dressing with an elastic bandage leaving the tips of the fingers free. Use elastic bandages only if the distal extremity is wrapped in continuity or edema will result distal to the bandage.

Most of the pain experienced after trauma to the hand results from edema. This can be alleviated by the moderate pressure provided by the elastic wrap, by providing the patient with a sling to keep the hand from being fully dependent, and by instructing the patient to keep the hand elevated on a pillow at night.

Excessive motion across a wound hinders healing. For this reason it is often wise to use a splint to limit motion and promote healing. This is especially important in wounds of the fingers and wrist. Some splinting can be obtained by using a bulky dressing. The easiest splints to use are the preformed aluminum or plastic splints. These are ideal for the fingers or the wrist. Though they are both strong and lightweight, they cannot always be used because of size limitations. In this event a lightweight splint can be fashioned out of 5 to 10 layers of plaster of Paris, molded for a perfect fit. Remove the splint as soon as it is no longer needed, or joint stiffness will result.

TETANUS PROPHYLAXIS

When treating acute wounds, the practitioner should always keep in mind the need for tetanus prophylaxis. The first and most important step in tetanus prophylaxis is meticulous wound care, including adequate debridement of devitalized tissue and removal of all foreign material. The guidelines for prophylaxis, though straightforward, should be individualized for each patient, consideration given to the characteristics of the wound, its age, and the conditions under which it occurred, as well as the immunization history of the patient.

Guidelines for tetanus prophylaxis

1. History of immunization or booster within 1 year—no therapy necessary
2. History of active immunization or booster within 1 to 5 years:
   a. Clean, minor wound—no antitetanus therapy needed
   b. Clean, major wound, tetanus prone—0.5 ml tetanus toxoid IM
   c. Contaminated wound, very tetanus prone—0.5 ml tetanus toxoid IM
3. History of immunization or booster within 5 to 10 years:
   a. Clean, minor wound—0.5 ml tetanus toxoid IM
   b. Clean, major wound, tetanus prone—0.5 ml tetanus toxoid IM
   c. Contaminated wound, very tetanus prone—0.5 ml tetanus toxoid IM plus antibotics

4. History of immunization or booster longer than 10 years:
   a. Clean, minor wound—0.5 ml tetanus toxoid IM
   b. Clean, major wound, tetanus prone—0.5 ml tetanus toxoid IM; 250 units human tetanus immunoglobulin
   c. Contaminated wound, very tetanus prone—0.5 ml tetanus toxoid IM, plus 250 units human tetanus immunoglobulin, and antibiotics
5. No history of complete immunization:
   a. Clean, minor wound—begin or complete immunization as per schedule (3 injections of 0.5 ml at 1-month intervals plus booster at 1 year)
   b. Clean, major wound, tetanus prone—0.5 ml tetanus toxoid IM and complete schedule plus 250 mg human tetanus immunoglobulin
   c. Contaminated wound, very tetanus prone—0.5 ml tetanus toxoid IM and complete schedule, plus 500 mg human tetanus immunoglobulin, and antibiotics

It is very important not to mix tetanus toxoid and immunoglobulin. They should be given with different syringes and needles and preferably at distant sites.

BITES
Animal bites

Though most animal bites are superficial and can be handled easily by the practitioner, some are disfiguring, with extensive tissue loss, and require the expertise of a trained surgeon. Small superficial wounds caused by a domestic animal, especially those of the face, may be closed loosely, provided the wound is observed daily.

The real decision to make regarding animal bites is whether or not to start antirabies therapy. Though in the past most cases of rabies resulted from bites of domestic animals, at the present time over half of the cases result from bites of wild animals.

Vaccination. One ml of human diploid cell rabies vaccine (HDCV) is given subcutaneously each day for 14 days. Start the series of inoculations 24 hours after rabies immune globulin has been administered. Booster injections are required at 10, 20, and 30 days following the initial course. Discontinue therapy if neurologic signs develop.

Table 5-1. Specific systemic treatment for rabies

Nature of exposure	Status of biting animal (vaccinated or not)		Recommended treatment
	At time of exposure	Ten-day observation period	
Lesion (indirect contact)	Rabid		None
Licks			
Unabraded skin	Rabid		None
Abraded skin, scratches, and unabraded or abraded mucosa	Healthy	Clinical signs of rabies or proved rabid (laboratory)	Start vaccine at first signs of rabies in biting animal
	Signs suggestive of rabies	Healthy	Start vaccine immediately; stop treatment if animal is normal on fifth day after exposure
	Rabid, escaped, killed, unknown		Start vaccine immediately
Bites			
Mild exposure	Healthy	Clinical signs of rabies or proved rabid (laboratory)	Start vaccine at first sign of rabies in biting animal
	Signs suggestive of rabies	Healthy	Start vaccine immediately; stop treatment if animal is normal on fifth day after exposure
	Rabid, escaped, killed, unknown		Start vaccine immediately
	Wild (wolf, jackal, fox, bat, etc.)		Serum immediately, followed by vaccine
Severe exposure (multiple or face, head, finger, or neck bites)	Healthy	Clinical signs of rabies or proved rabid (laboratory)	Serum immediately; start vaccine at first sign of rabies in biting animal

From WHO Expert Committee on Rabies, Technical Report Series, No. 321, 1966.

Table 5-1. Specific systemic treatment for rabies—cont'd

| Nature of exposure | Status of biting animal (vaccinated or not) | | Recommended treatment |
	At time of exposure	Ten-day ob-servation period	
Severe expo-sure—cont'd	Signs sugges-tive of rabies	Healthy	Serum immediate-ly, followed by vaccine; stop treatment if ani-mal is normal on fifth day after exposure
	Rabid, escaped, killed, unknown Wild (wolf, jackal, pariah dog, fox, bat, etc.)		Serum immediate-ly, followed by vaccine

Antiserum. Passive immunization with rabies immune globu-lin (RIG) is started as soon as possible. The usual dose is one vial: 1500 units in adults, or 300 units in children. Test the patient for sensitivity before injecting. If RIG is not available, use equine antirabies serum (1000 units/40kg body weight). Acceptable guidelines for the use of HDCV and RIG have been devel-oped by the World Health Organization and are given in Table 5-1.

Human bites

Human bites are the most potentially dangerous of all wounds. All such wounds should be considered contaminated and left open. Irrigate these wounds with copious amounts of normal saline or mild antiseptic solutions such as iodophor, wrap in a bulky dressing (Chapter 7), and observe daily for signs of infection.

THERMAL INJURY

The practitioner is frequently called on to care for minor thermal injury and should be prepared to offer emergency aid for major burns.

Evaluation of injury

The extent of thermal injury is expressed as a percentage of body surface. For rapid estimation, the Rule of Nines is employed (Table 5-2). This type of estimation is applicable only to adults because children have different body proportions. For a more accurate estimation of percent of surface burned and for record keeping, a burn chart such as that developed by the American College of Surgeons is necessary (Table 5-3).

The depth of burn injury is also useful in estimating the severity of the injury. *First degree burns* are characteristically hyperemic and hyperesthetic. *Second degree burns* (partial thickness) are superficial and erythematous. There is blister formation, or they are weeping and painful. *Third degree burns* (full thickness) are insensitive, and dry hard and translucent; and thrombosed veins are often visible.

Most mild first degree burns, such as sunburn, should be treated on an outpatient basis by instructing the patient to keep the wound clean with a mild soap solution. Avoid ointments and salves. Some severe first degree burns will require hospitalization.

Most minor second degree burns of less than 10% to 15% of body surface area can also be treated on an outpatient basis. Burns in infants and older adults, as well as burns of the hands, feet, face, and perineum, are of special significance and require the care of a trained physician unless extremely mild. Since the burn wound is open and easily contaminated, use strict aseptic techniques when evaluating the wound, including gloves, mask, and cap. After evaluation, cleanse the wound thoroughly with a mild soap solution and rinse well. Most surgeons recommend treating large blisters at this time, but small blisters should be left alone. If seen very early, these minor burns should then be treated with cold wet compresses. This therapy is effective in relieving pain and is indicated only if the burns are seen very early. Apply a topical antibiotic such as mafenide (Sulfamylon) or silver sulfadiazine and cover with a bulky dressing. Reexamine the wound the next day and, if all looks well, instruct the patient on cleansing and dressing the wound, and in the application of the antibiotic cream. Follow the progress at frequent intervals until healing is complete.

Table 5-2. Rule of nines

Region	Percent
Head and neck	9
Upper extremities	18 (9 × 2)
Lower extremities	36 (18 × 2)
Anterior surface of trunk	18
Posterior surface of trunk	18
Perineum	1
TOTAL	100

Table 5-3. Estimating percent of burn: relative percentages of areas affected by growth

Area	Age				
	Infant	1 to 4	5 to 9	10 to 14	Adult
Head	19	17	13	11	7
½ thigh	5½	6½	8	8½	9½
½ leg	5	5	5½	6	7

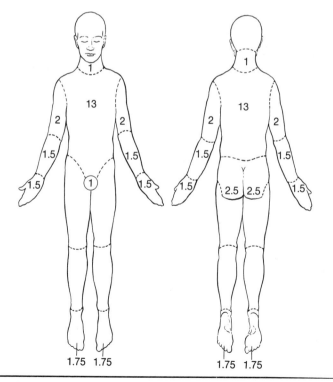

From Committee on Trauma, American College of Surgeons: A guide to initial therapy of burns, Chicago, 1974.

Though more severe burns are treated by trained surgeons, every practitioner should know the fundamentals of emergency care. Major burns are truly catastrophic with widespread systemic consequences. Direct your attention to these systemic problems first.

Emergency care at the scene

1. Stop the burning process.
2. Evaluate and maintain airway patency; check for respiratory burn or smoke inhalation.
3. Determine extent of burns (Rule of Nines); obtain history.
4. Prevent shock; start an intravenous infusion—burns less than 30%—500 ml of Ringer's lactate/hr (adult); burns more than 30%—1000 ml of Ringer's lactate/hr (adult). Do not start if within 30 minutes of a hospital.
5. Cover wounds with clean or sterile sheets, keep warm, do not use cool moist compresses.
6. Transport as soon as possible to a hospital.

Emergency management at the hospital

1. Call for assistance.
2. Check for adequate airway; intubate if necessary; avoid tracheostomy.
3. Prevention of shock.
   a. Evaluate previous IV lines, initiate new lines under optimal sterile conditions, and at optimal sites.
   b. Rule out other severe injuries.
   c. Insert a Foley catheter for urinary output measurement. Maintain urinary output at a level of 50 ml/hr.
   d. Insert a nasogastric tube.
   e. Compute and start IV therapy; give 3 ml of Ringer's lactate for each percent of burn and for every kg of body weight (3 ml × _____% × _____ kg = _____). Plan to give half of this amount in the first 8 hours.
   f. Once resuscitation is underway and the patient's vital signs are stable, Demerol or morphine may be given IV (do *not* give IM because of irregular absorption).
   g. Start tetanus prophylaxis if needed.

h. Cleanse wound with a mild soap solution.

i. Surrender care to a primary physician as soon as one arrives.

Before attempting any closure, remember to make sure that the wound is free of foreign material, that all devitalized tissue has been removed, and that adequate hemostasis has been obtained either by ligation with absorbable suture or by electrosurgical coagulation.

Delayed primary closure is a useful technique in dealing with moderately contaminated wounds or wounds more than 8 hours old. After thorough cleansing and debridement, pack the wound with a mild antiseptic soaked gauze (such as iodophor) and, if at 4 days the wound looks clean and there is no evidence of infection, close the wound loosely. Sometimes sutures can be placed at the time of debridement and tied down later, avoiding the necessity of a second anesthesia.

For more grossly contaminated and infected wounds it is best to leave the wound open for adequate drainage and to allow healthy granulation tissue to cover the wound (Chapter 6). Once granulation is complete, usually at about 2 weeks, closure can be attempted.

SUTURE REMOVAL

The length of time sutures are needed varies according to the rapidity of wound healing. This depends partly on vascularity and tendency toward edema. Different areas heal at different rates. Leave sutures in until the wound is well healed. The following general guidelines should be noted:

Face and neck	4 to 5 days
Trunk	7 to 10 days
Upper extremities and hands	10 to 12 days
Lower extremities and feet	12 to 16 days

6

Care of the chronic and infected wound and treatment of infections

Many wounds require prolonged care, such as contaminated wounds that are left open for treatment, chronic skin ulcers, and burns. Therefore the practitioner needs to become acquainted with the surgical principles involved in their care.

CHRONIC WOUNDS

To treat chronic wounds on an outpatient basis, the full co-operation of the patient must be enlisted and the wound should be checked on a regular basis. If there is no evidence of improvement or healing, seek more professional advice. It is amazing how quickly some chronic wounds heal once the patient is admitted to the hospital.

As a general rule, use moist compresses if the wound exudes a copious amount of material or has a thick, tenacious coagulum at the base. The principle involved is to keep the exudate liquid and, by capillary action within the dressing, to "wick" it away from the wound base. Normal saline solution works fine for this purpose, or a mild antibacterial agent such as half-strength Betadine or Dakin's solution can be used. Because the task is to loosen and remove the exudate, the dressing should be changed frequently: at least three times a day. The technique is extremely simple and can usually be performed by the patient. Merely soak a sufficient number of gauze sponges in normal saline solution or mild antiseptic and apply to the wound, trying to fill all crevices. Hold this compress in place with elasticized cotton rolls such as Kerlix or elastic netting. On the distal extremities, an elastic bandage is particularly helpful. If the gauze packing tends to dry out too rapidly, a piece of plastic or Saran Wrap placed over the sponges will help retain the moisture. If the wound is located on an extremity, the patient should keep the extremity elevated as much as possible.

A useful technique for debridement of tenacious coagulum or eschar is the wet-to-dry dressing. This is similar to the wet compress, but the compress is not as saturated and dries out within 4 hours. The coagulum then dries within the interstices of the gauze, so that when the gauze is removed, it takes with it some of the coagulum and eschar. This is less effective as an outpatient treatment because it is sometimes painful and the patient often avoids dressing changes. For especially tenacious eschars, chemical debriding agents, such as Travase or Elase, are effective. These dissolve the eschar by enzymatic breakdown.

Because of associated swelling and edema, chronic wounds of the lower extremity are often helped by compression and immobilization. An elastic wrap is often helpful. In more chronic indolent wounds a Gelocast or Unna boot often proves effective, especially for venous stasis ulcers. An Unna boot consists of gauze impregnated with zinc oxide and calamine. It provides moderate compression and immobilization plus protective emollients for adjacent tissues. The Unna boot should be changed weekly.

When all else fails, a regular cast of plaster or fiberglass will often promote rapid healing. The cast can be "windowed" to allow for local wound care.

The outpatient treatment of minimal to mild second degree burns can be accomplished by following similar guidelines. After initial therapy, the patient should be instructed in the outpatient care of the wound. The wound should be cleansed two to three times a day with a mild soap solution, then a layer of silver sulfadiazine about 1/8 inch thick should be applied. This is then covered with a layer of fine mesh gauze. The dressing is protected with several additional layers of gauze and is held in place with Kerlix or elastic net. If the gauze sticks to the wound during dressing changes, the innermost layer may be soaked off.

The chronic wound should be observed routinely to ensure the progression of the healing process. Most chronic wounds are considered "contaminated" and the use of antibiotics is not routinely necessary. Their use should be considered in dirty wounds, chronic wounds newly presented for therapy, and wounds that do not respond to more conservative therapy, unlike acute wounds.

Chronic wounds are often colonized by gram-negative bacteria, making sensitivity testing extremely important for appropriate antibiotic choice. Until sensitivity results are available, antibiotics of choice include wide-spectrum cephalosporins, aminoglycosides and the newer synthetic penicillins. Selection of the appropriate antibiotic should be predicated on sensitivity testing.

More indolent wounds, especially of the lower extremity, are often colonized with fungi—typically *Candida Albicans*. Gentian violet applied topically is often effective in treating this superficial contamination.

Failure of the chronic wound to respond to adequate therapy or deterioration in spite of therapy signifies that more experienced professional help is needed.

INFECTED WOUNDS

The diagnosis of surgical infection, abscess, and/or cellulitis should be considered when the following criteria are met:

Tumor—mass, edema
Calor—heat
Rubor—redness, erythema
Dolor—pain

Though these descriptive terms date back to the early days of surgery, they are still accurate. Wounds that continue to exude purulent material should be added to this list, as well as patients with chronic wounds who become febrile.

Most wound infections begin as a cellulitis, a nonlocalized infection in the skin and subcutaneous layers. If cellulitis is treated in its early phase with appropriate antibiotics, its progression toward localization and abscess formation can be halted. The typical cellulitis is often caused by streptococcal infections, and the treatment of choice is penicillin, rest, and the application of local heat, with surgical drainage delayed until collections of pus become evident. Most cellulitis occurring around primarily closed wounds represents the early stages of a staphylococcal infection with rapid progression to pus formation and the production of an abscess.

The only adequate treatment of an abscess is adequate surgical drainage. In infected primarily closed wounds, this means that the sutures should be removed and, if the wound does not open by itself, the wound margins should be spread gently with a hemostat at the point of maximal erythema and tenderness. If this does not produce drainage and no fluctuance is evident (a soft area amidst the more indurated tissue), administer antibiotics, provide rest, and apply moist compresses to the area. If there is some question as to the presence of fluctuance, needle aspiration will help in the diagnosis. Check the wound at frequent intervals until there is clear evidence of improvement or until suppuration is evident, at which time the wound should be drained.

If the wound does not open upon removal of the stitches and gentle prodding, and if fluctuance is present, drain the wound at this time. This usually requires local anesthesia, which is best provided by field or regional block. The abscess and adjacent areas are acutely tender and infected, so it is best not to use infiltration techniques. After anesthesia has been administered, separate the wound edges with a hemostat or divide with a scalpel directly over the area of fluctuance. Obtain a sample of the exudate for culture and sensitivity studies. Separate the wound margins as widely as possible and loosely pack the wound to keep the edges separated. Apply a dry sterile dressing.

Since most staphylococcal infections in primarily closed wounds are caused by penicillin-resistant staphylococci, the patient should be given a semisynthetic penicillin (such as methicillin or oxacillin) pending the results of the sensitivity tests. Ancillary therapy includes elevation, if an extremity is involved, rest, and frequent dressing changes following adequate drainage.

Check the wound in 24 to 48 hours and remove the packing. The packing should be replaced if the cavity remains large or if there continues to be a large amount of exudate. Repack at 48- to 72-hour intervals until adequate healing is ensured.

Do not pack abscess cavities tightly. This inhibits the free flow of exudate and hinders the obliteration of the cavity, which results from contraction of the wound edges and cavity walls. The main purpose of the pack is to facilitate drainage and to keep the skin edges from healing over before the abscess cavity is obliterated. Packing should be loose and some of the packing should protrude from the wound onto the skin. Use small packing strips (such as Nu-Gauz). These can be soaked first in a mild antibiotic or an antiseptic solution such as Betadine.

If a patient complains of increasing pain at the site of the wound, or develops systemic signs such as fever and chills, check the wound immediately. This usually means infection. Particularly severe infections that every practitioner should be aware of are clostridial myositis (gas gangrene) and clostridial cellulitis. These infections usually develop in extensive wounds with significant devitalization of tissue that has been grossly contaminated.

The average incubation period for clostridial myositis is 48 hours. The first clinical manifestation is pain. The skin around the wound is pale, shiny, and edematous. A brownish, watery discharge with a foul odor is usually present. Crepitus is usually a late finding. Systemic symptoms develop rapidly with a rapid, feeble pulse being predominant and out of line with the febrile response. As the infection progresses, the patient has difficulty maintaining blood pressure and appears extremely ill. This infection requires the services of a fully trained surgeon for wide debridement and possible amputation.

Clostridial cellulitis involves fascia and connective tissue, with development of crepitus. The onset of this infection is more gradual than myositis and begins about 3 to 4 days after injury. Though less toxic systemically than myositis, the tissue destruction can be extensive. The necessary debridement requires the care of a surgeon.

INFECTIONS TREATED SURGICALLY

The practitioner is often called on to treat surgical infections not arising in conjunction with wounds. The treatment principles are generally the same.

Cellulitis as a nonlocalized infection in the subcutaneous layer is ordinarily well conrolled by antibiotics. Surgical intervention is usually not necessary. Often this infection is associated with lymphangitis and diagnosed by redness and inflammation along the lymph channels, usually in the extremities. This type of infection should also respond to antibiotic therapy. If the infection reaches the lymph nodes, lymphadenitis will result. In the early stages antibiotic therapy is adequate, but if suppuration and fluctuance occur, surgical drainage becomes mandatory.

Most abscesses start as relatively superficial infections at the base of hair follicles and are called furuncles or folliculitis. These usually remain small and well localized and, because of their superficial location, rupture early and drain spontaneously so that little has to be done surgically. If they burrow deeply, however, they become true abscesses and must be drained surgically. Prepare the area as for any other formal surgical procedure and anesthetize the area. If these abscesses are quite deep, infiltrate the line of the proposed incision with a small amount of anesthetic directly over the abscess. If the abscess is very superficial, topical ethyl chloride should be adequate. Insert a No. 11 blade into the abscess at one side and withdraw it in a sweeping motion to completely incise the roof of the abscess (Fig. 6-1). Spread the wound margins with a hemostat and obtain a specimen for culture and sensitivity. Then proceed as with any other abscess.

A particularly severe type of abscess is the carbuncle. This is usually seen in diabetic patients, often on the nape of the neck, and represents an abscess that involves many hair follicles and, therefore, has many loculations. To adequately treat a carbuncle, all these loculations have to be broken up. This requires a cruciate incision over the area and surgical disruption of the collections of pus (Fig. 6-2). Patients with carbuncles are often diabetic and the infection is severe, treatment often requires hospitalization.

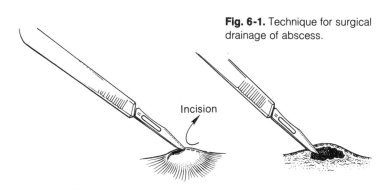

Fig. 6-1. Technique for surgical drainage of abscess.

Incision

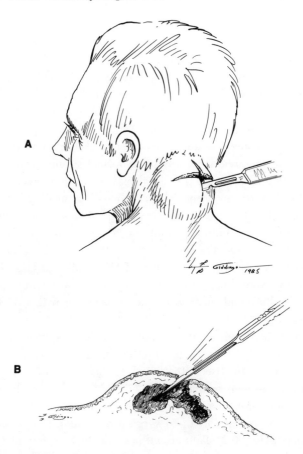

Fig. 6-2. A, Technique of cruciate incision for drainage of a carbuncle. **B,** Technique for breaking up loculations within a carbuncle.

Another important and dangerous abscess is the felon. This is an abscess in the pad at the tip of the finger. This is a closed space because of the anatomic arrangement of the distal phalanx. An infection with edema and pus formation can increase pressure enough to cause ischemia and necrosis or permanent nerve damage. Because of this pressure, it is also extremely painful. It is also somewhat like a carbuncle in that the numerous fascial bands that honeycomb the fat pad cause numerous loculations. To effectively treat this lesion, a through-and-through incision under re-

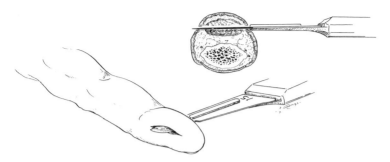

Fig. 6-3. Technique for surgical drainage of a felon.

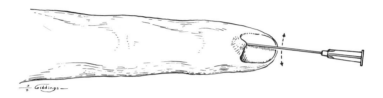

Fig. 6-4. Technique for drainage of a paronychia.

gional anesthesia is made through the fat pad close to the bone and a small wick is placed through this tract (Fig. 6-3). Felons are best treated by a trained surgeon.

Another abscess that deserves attention is the perirectal abscess. Though this can start as a folliculitis and furuncle, it usually signifies a deep abscess originating from the crypts within the rectum. If small and obviously superficial, these abscesses can be treated as outlined previously; otherwise these patients should be hospitalized and under the care of a surgeon.

A paronychia is an infection of the tissue surrounding the fingernail and, if left unattended, can result in the destruction of the nail bed or develop into a felon. Because these are very superficial, they are easily treated, usually without anesthesia. After adequate preparation of the area, gently elevate the cuticle of the nail until the collection is entered (Fig. 6-4). Instruct the patient to soak the hand twice a day in a warm, mild soap solution.

Epidermoid and pilonidal cysts often become infected. Once infected, they should be treated as abscesses and drained. Do not try to excise the cysts while infection is still present.

Acute infections, not acquired in the hospital, are usually caused by a penicillin-sensitive *Staphylococcus aureus*. Penicillin or a first generation cephalosporin is the antibiotic of choice until appropriate sensitivity studies are obtained.

7

Intravenous techniques

Over a century ago, Scotland was swept by an epidemic of cholera. During that period Thomas Latta, a physician of Leith, discovered that cholera kills by dehydration. He managed to save several victims by dissolving mineral salts in water and infusing the mixture into their veins. After this crude beginning, intravenous infusion therapy is now used in virtually every branch of medicine. Much has been written on intravenous fluid therapy, detailing with great precision what should be given and why it should be given. This chapter has a more modest aim: to outline how to gain access to the venous circulation.

PERIPHERAL VENIPUNCTURE

A number of devices are used for peripheral venipuncture. The straight, hollow needle was standard for many years. It has been replaced by the butterfly needle, a descendent of the scalp vein needle used in infants, and by through-needle and over-needle catheters (Fig. 7-1). Each device requires a slightly different insertion technique. Venipuncture technique will be described with a straight needle, with a butterfly needle, and then with the other forms.

In a venous cannulation the longevity of a site is ultimately limited by the tendency of the vein to thrombose under the influence of whatever fluids are being administered. However, in practice, most intravenous sites become unusable as a result of the cannula pulling out, perforating the back wall of the vein, or causing thrombosis by mechanical or chemical irritation. Any insertion technique must therefore achieve not only placement of the cannula but also proper fixation to prevent subsequent dislodgment or excessive movement of the cannula.

The first step in inserting a cannula of any kind is to select a site. Nine times out of ten the site will be in the forearm or the back of the hand. The veins there are large and easily seen even

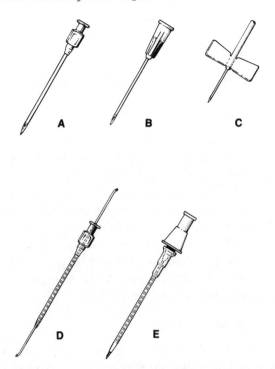

Fig. 7-1. Tools of venous access: **A** and **B,** straight, hollow needles, **C,** butterfly needle, **D,** through-needle catheter, and, **E,** over-needle catheter. Each of these is available from different manufacturers with minor variations.

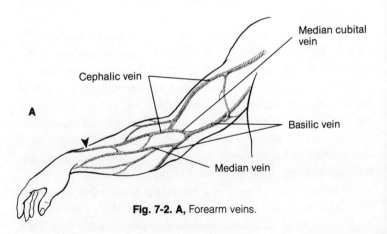

Fig. 7-2. A, Forearm veins.

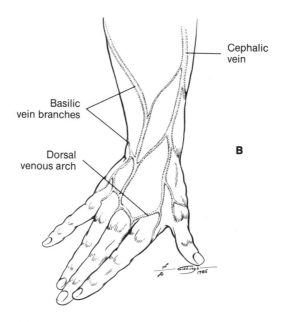

Fig. 7-2, cont'd. B, Hand veins. These are easy to see, rarely covered with fat, and relatively strong. Notice the large cephalic vein at the distal, radial portion of forearm.

in obese people, and cannulas can be secured easily (Fig. 7-2). Probably the best single site in the body is the cephalic vein, located about 10 cm above the wrist (Fig. 7-2, A). The large median cubital vein in the antecubital fossa would seem to be ideal, however, the motion of the elbow makes it almost impossible to fix a cannula adequately.

The scalp veins are universally used in infants, since they are relatively large and located just beneath the thin skin of the scalp. Special scalp vein sets, which are butterfly needles of 23, 25, or 27 gauge, are used. Actually, cannulating the vein is simple compared with fixing the cannula. The fixation technique often involves placing cotton balls under the butterfly wings to fix the needle at the proper angle and using large amounts of adhesive tape to secure it.

Lower extremity veins should be used only as a last resort, although the dorsal veins of the foot are easy to cannulate, and

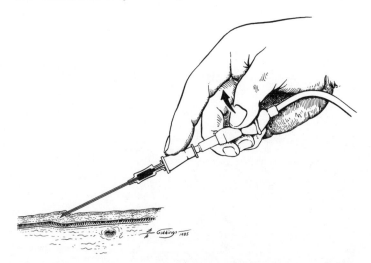

Fig. 7-3. Technique of needle puncture of the vein. Notice that the needle has been placed through the skin first and will be placed through the vein subsequently.

the saphenous vein is near the surface and quite easy to find. There is a real risk of causing thrombosis of the leg veins and perhaps pulmonary emboli.

After the site has been chosen, the skin should be prepared. The common practice is to use an alcohol swab; this smells good but is ineffectual (see Chapter 1). A more effective method is to use an iodophor solution.

Take an 18- or 20-gauge needle, and place it either on the end of the intravenous tubing (Fig. 7-3) or on the end of a syringe. Experts disagree over which is better, but both are effective. Place the needle along the vein, flat on the skin, bevel up, with the point a few millimeters from the proposed site of venous entry. If using the needle on intravenous tubing, squeeze a few drops of fluid out of the needle with the bulb in the tubing. Puncture the skin. Next release the bulb, or put a little suction on the needle, so that entry into the vein will be indicated by a blood return in the needle. Then, puncture the vein. Most beginners try to puncture the skin and the vein in one motion; this rarely works. Advance the needle into the vein; ideally, the hub should be against the skin puncture site. Stabilize the needle with tape (Fig. 7-4) and secure a loop of tubing to the skin to prevent the tubing from pulling on the needle.

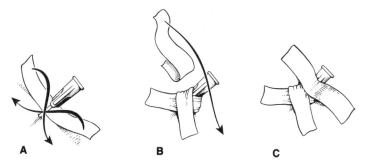

Fig. 7-4. Technique of securing needle to the skin.

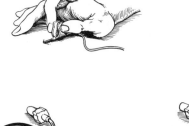

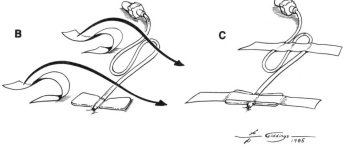

Fig. 7-5. A, Technique of inserting butterfly needle and, **B** and **C,** securing butterfly needle to skin.

Inserting a butterfly needle uses a similar technique (Fig. 7-5). Butterfly needles range in size from 16 to 27 gauge; the size should be chosen to fit the vein. Usually, a 19 or 21 gauge is best. The plastic butterfly wings, folded together, are a convenient bundle. The skin should be punctured first, then the vein. If the end of the tubing attached to the needle is left open, blood will flow back to signal entry into the vein. The butterfly wings can be taped to the skin, providing much better fixation than is possible with a straight needle (Fig. 7-5). A loop of the tubing should be taped to the skin.

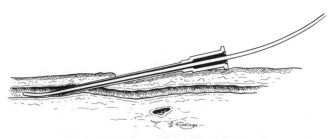

Fig. 7-6. Insertion of through-needle catheter.

The through-needle catheters allow passage of a Teflon or polyethylene catheter into the vein for several centimeters; however, the technique of insertion is more difficult. Place the needle into the vein in the usual manner. Advance the catheter through the needle into the vein (Fig. 7-6). Then withdraw the needle. Inserting these catheters presents two problems. First, the needle must be bigger than the catheter; hence, a rather large needle must be used. Because the catheters are long, a 14- or 16-gauge catheter must be used to allow adequate flow. This means using a 12- or 14-gauge needle. Large needles are difficult to place and make holes in the vein which are larger than the catheter; this makes the procedure somewhat bloody. The second problem is what to do with the needle. If the needle is left in place over the catheter it may cut the catheter, and lead to catheter embolus. There have been quite a number of such emboli over the past few years. Although the techniques of extracting them are of great interest to cardiologists and cardiac surgeons, it is best to avoid the problem by removing the needle. This means, however, that the catheter hub must be detachable which in turn means that it may become dislodged later on, thus creating the risk of air embolus.

Over-needle catheters were designed to solve both of these problems. These units are available in both Teflon and polyethylene, with permanently attached hubs, in sizes from 14 to 20 gauge. The 14- and 16-gauge catheters are probably the most commonly used. The needle and catheter together are inserted in a manner similar to that used with a straight needle (Fig. 7-7). Then the needle is withdrawn, leaving the catheter in the vein, and the intravenous tubing is connected to the catheter hub. Taping is the same as for a needle. The pliant catheter will not puncture the vein, and the length ensures that it will not be

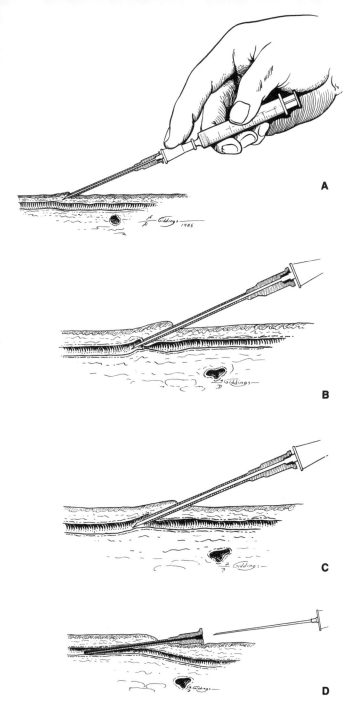

Fig. 7-7. Insertion of the over-needle catheter. In **A,** the needle and catheter have been inserted through the skin. In **B,** the needle tip has been inserted into the vein. Blood can be aspirated, but the catheter is not yet in the vein. The tip of the needle must be raised to avoid impaling the back wall and the needle must be advanced further to carry the catheter into the vein as in **C.** In **D,** the needle is removed and the catheter threaded into the vein.

dislodged if the skin fixation is adequate. The only major drawback is that over-needle catheters are more difficult to insert than either straight needles or butterfly needles. A close view of the tip of the device as it passes into the vein shows the problem (Fig. 7-7, *B*). The needle has punctured the vein and blood can be aspirated through it, but the catheter is larger than the hole in the vein and is not yet in the vein. Tilt the needle up and push the catheter into the vein. Do not push the needle through the back wall of the vein.

As a general recommendation, the butterfly needle is probably best for the dorsum of the hand and the over-needle catheter for the forearm veins. Most situations can be handled satisfactorily by one or the other.

CENTRAL VENOUS TECHNIQUES

Although peripheral venipuncture is satisfactory for most intravenous infusions, it is sometimes necessary to gain access to the central veins. Three indications for this are central venous pressure measurement, total parenteral nutrition, and unavailability of other access sites.

Central venous pressure measurement is usually performed by connecting a saline manometer to a catheter with the tip in the superior vena cava. Central venous pressure is a somewhat unreliable, but often useful, guide to the patient's fluid status; if a patient is hypovolemic, the pressure will be low and will remain low until the patient has a normal volume of circulating fluid. It is less accurate as a guide to the volume status than is the left atrial pressure, or the pulmonary capillary wedge pressure, which will be discussed later in the section on pulmonary artery catheters.

The hypertonic glucose solutions used in total parenteral nutrition administration will damage peripheral veins, producing thrombosis of the veins within hours. These solutions must be given into the central veins so that the hypertonic fluid is diluted by the greater blood flow around the catheter.

Four types of catheter sets are available for central venous access. In the simplest type (Fig. 7-8), a 7- to 8-cm straight needle is used to puncture the subclavian vein and a catheter is passed through it. The needle is completely removed and a hub is attached to the catheter. This is fast and easy, but the catheter-to-hub junction is critical. If it comes apart later, the patient may

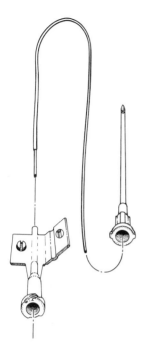

Fig. 7-8. Straight catheter through needle.

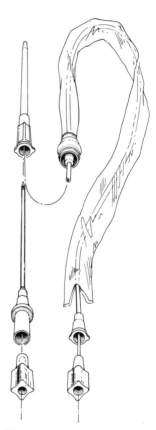

Fig. 7-9. Catheter through an over-needle catheter.

develop an air embolism. The second type uses an over-needle cannula (Fig. 7-9). Once the vein is entered, the needle is removed and the central venous catheter is passed through the over-needle catheter. In this way a central venous catheter with a molded hub can be used, but the over-needle catheter has to stay in place.

Fig. 7-10. Catheter over guidewire.

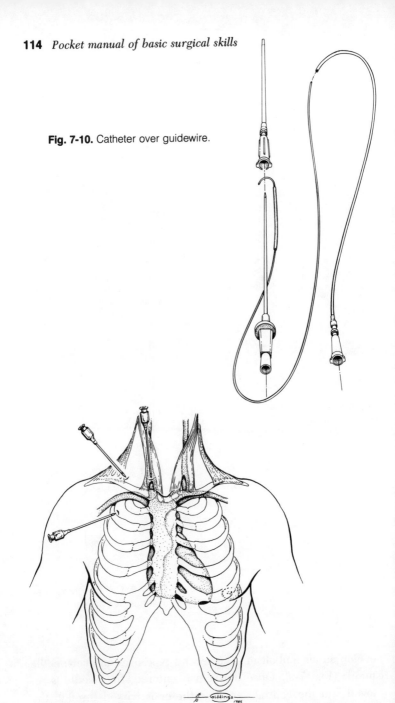

Fig. 7-11. Sites of access to the central veins: infraclavicular, supraclavicular, and internal jugular (between the sternal and clavicular heads of the sternocleidomastoid muscle).

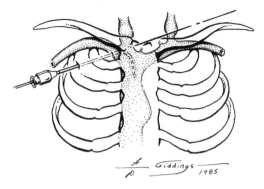

Fig. 7-12. Infraclavicular access.

The other two types of catheter sets are designed to avoid leaving the over-needle catheter in place. The third type uses a guidewire (Fig. 7-10), which can be placed through a needle or an over-needle catheter. All but the guidewire is removed and the central venous catheter is passed over the guidewire. The fourth type uses a "peel-away" type of over-needle catheter passed over a guidewire. This type is used for passing Silastic catheter for chronic access. The technique is described later.

The subclavian vein may be reached by either a supraclavicular or an infraclavicular approach. The internal jugular vein may be reached through the neck. All of these approaches have their advocates and each presents certain hazards (Fig. 7-11).

Infraclavicular approach

Place the patient in the Trendelenburg position to fill the veins and prevent air emboli. Prepare the skin meticulously with iodophor. Use drapes, gloves, and mask. Place a pad under the patient's shoulder to lift the clavicle, widening the space between it and the first rib. After raising a skin wheal with a local anesthetic, use a No. 11 blade to place a small puncture wound in the skin of the chest approximately 5 cm below the midpoint of the clavicle (Fig. 7-12). This allows entry of the needle without friction at the skin puncture site. Attach a syringe to the needle and direct the needle toward the hollow just above the manubrium. Usually, the clavicle will be encountered first. Withdraw the needle slightly and direct it deep toward the clavicle while aspirating on the syringe. If all goes well, the needle will enter the subclavian vein and blood will aspirate freely. If not, withdraw the needle completely, reevaluate the landmarks, and try again. If you still fail, find someone with more experience, since this is not a procedure in which persistence pays off. The vein tends to contract and presents a smaller target, therefore the complication rate rises markedly with repeated attempts.

When the needle is in the vein, grasp the hub with a large hemostat to secure it and take off the syringe. Blood should flow from the needle because the patient is in the head-down position. If it does not, put the syringe back on immediately. Air can be sucked in through the needle into the central veins, and even a small air embolus can be fatal. Then advance the catheter through the needle. If the catheter does not advance, *do not* pull it back through the needle. Pulling a catheter back in this situation may cause it to be sheared off by the sharp needle tip. Advance the catheter so that its tip is in the mid-superior vena cava and withdraw the needle over the catheter.

For the over-needle catheter, advance the catheter over the needle, and into the vein. Remove the needle. Then place the central catheter through the over-needle catheter.

If using a guidewire, pass it through the needle. Advance the needle. Then place the central venous catheter over the guidewire.

Supraclavicular approach

With the patient in the Trendelenburg position, prepare the skin over the clavicle. The site of puncture is 1 centimeter above the mid-portion of the clavicle (Fig. 7-13). Direct the needle about 30 degrees posteriorly and toward the opposite nipple. The "target" is the confluence of the subclavian vein and the internal jugular vein, which is deep to the sternomanubrial joint.

Internal jugular approach

Again, the patient is in Trendelenburg position, the skin prepared and drapes applied. There are three approaches: anterior

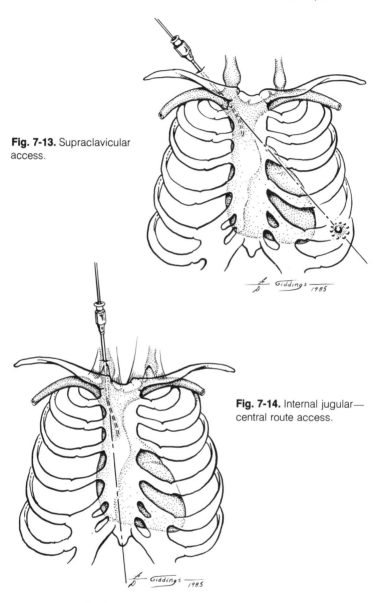

Fig. 7-13. Supraclavicular access.

Fig. 7-14. Internal jugular—central route access.

to the sternocleidomastoid muscle, posterior to it, and between the sternal and clavicular heads. This last is the "central" route and is the easiest of the three to achieve (Fig. 7-14). Identify the sternal and clavicular heads of the sternocleidomastoid. The puncture site is between them. Direct the needle 30 degrees posteriorly and aim toward the xiphoid process. The objective is to pierce the internal jugular vein just above its confluence with the subclavian vein.

Fixation of the central venous catheter is very important (Fig. 7-15). Take a suture in the skin, wrap it several times around the catheter, and tie it. Tape the hub of the catheter separately, looping the catheter to allow taping it to the skin of the chest. Secure the intravenous tubing. After placing iodophor ointment around the catheter entry site, cover with an occlusive sterile dressing. Catheter infections can be prevented by meticulous dressing technique because the usual route for infection is along the catheter tract. The dressing should be changed regularly,

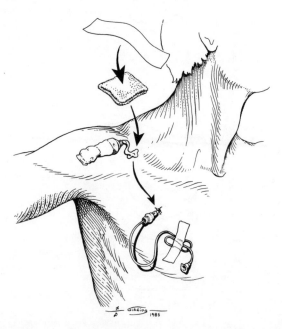

Fig. 7-15. Dressing and securing of the central venous catheter. Secure the catheter at the exit site with an extra suture. Tape the catheter and loop of intravenous tubing to the chest wall. Dress the entry site with iodophor ointment and an occlusive dressing. Use the same technique with the supra-clavicular and jugular routes. The central venous catheter is shown passing through an over-needle catheter, which can be left through the skin. When passing the central catheter through a needle, pull the needle free of the skin, and secure the catheter to the skin between the end of the needle and the skin entry site; or, if possible, remove the needle entirely.

every 24 to 48 hours, after cleaning the skin surrounding the catheter and placement of iodophor ointment around the entry site.

There are several complications with this procedure, some of which may be fatal. Air embolization occurs when the catheter hub comes off or the tubing becomes disconnected. Pneumothorax may occur if the needle punctures the pleura and enters the underlying lung. Mediastinal hematoma may be caused by an unsuccessful puncture or by puncturing the back wall of the vein. The catheter may be advanced into the heart and cause arrhythmias or, more seriously, perforation and pericardial tamponade from infused fluid.

Immediately after the procedure an x-ray film of the chest should be obtained with a portable unit. The catheter should be clearly visible with the tip of the catheter positioned in the midpoint of the superior vena cava; if it is too far in, it should be pulled back (unless using a through-needle catheter, see discussion on p. 116).

The technique of subclavian puncture is useful and necessary, but it can be overused and is certainly dangerous. It should be performed only when absolutely necessary and with great care by an experienced individual.

LONG-TERM CENTRAL VENOUS ACCESS

Continuing access to the central veins is necessary for long-term parenteral nutrition. It is useful for cancer chemotherapy and for chronic antibiotic therapy. The usual polyethylene or Teflon catheter tends to cause too much reaction, leading to subclavian thrombosis. Silastic catheters, however, can be left in place for months or even years. Both single- and double-lumen catheters are available in several sizes.

Placing a Silastic catheter requires special technique. It is too flexible to pass over a guidewire. The problem is similar to placement of transvenous pacemaker leads and has been solved in the same way. Originally cutdown on the cephalic vein at the shoulder was used. But with development of the "peel-away" sheath, direct puncture has been the standard method.

The major drawback to long-term access is catheter-related infection. The tissue never heals to the catheter. A sheath of fibrous tissue forms around the catheter and between the catheter and the sheath is a space. Within the vein a thin fibrin sleeve forms around the catheter, so there is a direct tract from the entry site on the skin all the way to the tip of the catheter. The existence of this pathway poses a constant threat of infection. Meticulous dressing technique prevents infection in short-term catheter placement. But for long-term placement, more protection is needed. Long-term catheters are made with a Dacron felt ring attached, into which tissue grows. With the ring placed under the skin the continuity of the peri-catheter tract is broken and the risk of infection much diminished (Fig. 7-16). Of course, careful dressing technique is still necessary.

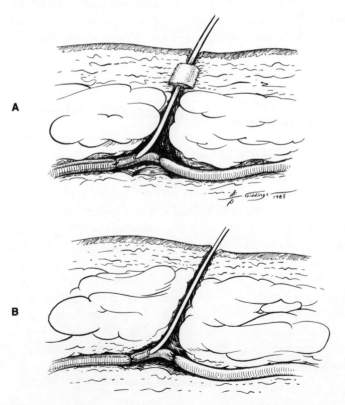

Fig. 7-16. Drawing of catheter sheath, **A,** with Dacron felt cuff, and, **B,** without cuff.

The catheter can be implanted by cephalic cutdown or by direct puncture. Both techniques will be described.

Cephalic cutdown. The cephalic vein is located in the deltopectoral groove (Fig. 7-17). Make a transverse incision in the skin of the shoulder, dissect down to the muscle, and try to find the groove, which can be difficult. Often one or two small venous tributaries will serve as guides to the cephalic vein. Even so the vein is inconstant and may be impossible to find. Measure the catheter and cut it to length. Thread the catheter into the cephalic vein using standard venous cutdown techniques. Then make a second incision, about 0.5 cm long medially over the pectoral muscle. Using a small clamp to hold the catheter, tunnel under the skin to the first incision and pull the catheter hub through. If the catheter length is correct, the Dacron felt cuff will be 2 to 3 cm from the exit site. Close both incisions. The felt cuff will fix the catheter adequately for long-term use but in the meantime a temporary fixation suture should be used.

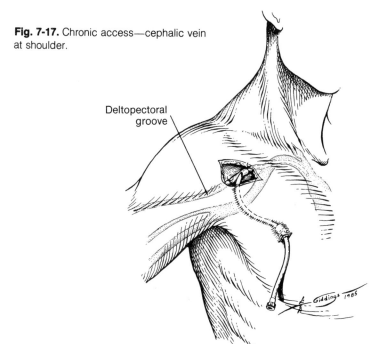

Fig. 7-17. Chronic access—cephalic vein at shoulder.

Deltopectoral groove

Placement with "peel-away" sheath. Position the patient for an infraclavicular approach: 15 degrees head-down, with the shoulder elevated on a rolled towel. Cut the catheter to fit by placing it on the skin over the projected course, and with the Dacron felt cuff 2 cm from the projected exit site. The catheter tip should lie in the vena cava, near the cava-atrial junction, which is under the midpoint of the sternum. Make a 2 cm transverse incision 5 cm below the midpoint of the clavicle. Then make a 0.5 mm incision at the proposed exit site. Tunnel a clamp from the larger incision to the exit incision. Pull the catheter, tip first, through the tunnel. Then pull it all the way through to have enough catheter to perform the cannulation.

Now proceed with the puncture. Direct the needle beneath the clavicle toward the hollow just above the manubrium. Puncture the vein. Pass the guidewire and remove the needle. Advance the sheath and dilator assembly over the guidewire. Remember, the sheath is fragile and may be difficult to pass under the clavicle, but a straight passage is essential. If the sheath curves around the clavicle, it will kink and the catheter will not pass through it. Sometimes re-puncture is necessary.

If passage of the sheath is impossible, divide the pectoral muscle and locate the brachial vein beneath it. Expose the vein and puncture it under direct vision. Pass the sheath and dilator over the guidewire.

Once the sheath is within the vein, remove the dilator and pass the Silastic catheter. There should be back-bleeding from the sheath. After the catheter is passed, aspirate to verify its position. Then grasp the "wings" of the sheath, one in each hand. Pull them straight apart, splitting the sheath down the middle, and remove the two halves. Take care not to remove the catheter during this procedure. Pull the catheter out, under the skin site positioning the Dacron felt ring 2 cm under the skin from the exit site. Close both incisions. A fixation suture may be temporarily placed to secure the felt ring to the skin.

Subsequent care of the catheter requires an occlusive dressing re-applied every 2 or 3 days. A popular technique is to use a plastic adhesive membrane (Op-site, for example) after applying a bit of iodophor ointment to the exit site. When not in use, the catheter should be filled with heparin saline solution (100 u/ml).

FEMORAL VENIPUNCTURE

The major purpose for femoral venipuncture is drawing blood from a patient who has no other access sites. Rarely, one needs to gain access to the circulation in an emergency and the femoral vein is convenient. A catheter should not be left in the femoral vein for more than a day because of the danger of deep venous thrombosis. The femoral route is often used for cardiac catheterization and for radiologic procedures.

The femoral vein is located just medial to the femoral artery in the groin (Fig. 7-18). Use a 18-gauge, 1½ inch needle, attached to a large syringe. While wearing gloves, prepare the skin with iodophor, palpate the femoral artery, and puncture the skin about 1 cm medial to the arterial pulse. With one finger on the femoral pulse, advance the needle perpendicular to the skin, medial to the artery, while aspirating on the syringe. If bone is

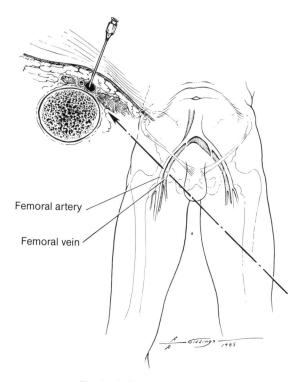

Femoral artery

Femoral vein

Fig. 7-18. Femoral puncture site.

reached, withdraw the needle, still aspirating. When blood is obtained, hold the needle in place 6 and draw the sample, then withdraw the needle and keep pressure on the site for 5 minutes. The major complication is mistakenly entering the artery. If this happens, draw the sample, remove the needle, and keep pressure on the site for 10 minutes. Then apply a pressure dressing by putting a large pad over the artery, then holding it in place with 2-inch tape from the inside of the thigh, over the iliac crest, to the lateral aspect of the flank.

VENOUS CUTDOWN

Open venous cannulation, or venous cutdown, is used for direct access to the peripheral veins for infusion catheters, cardiac catheterization, placement of pacemakers, central venous catheters, and emergency access. As with venipuncture the first step is to decide where access should be.

The most commonly used cutdown site is the brachial vein just above the elbow crease (Fig. 7-2). Any of the arm veins can be used for cutdown but this is the largest. It also allows direct cannulation of the central veins.

The cephalic vein is sometimes used (Fig. 7-17). The vein is inconstant but it can be used when implanting cardiac pacemakers and for situations in which the arm veins are not accessible.

The external jugular vein is commonly used (Fig. 7-19). This vein can be punctured percutaneously or aproached by cutdown. Place the incision directly over the vein. Tunnel the catheter under the skin for 5 or 6 cm, bringing the catheter out through a stab wound in the skin. Then cannulate the vein and close the incision. In this way the entry site is protected and the chance of late catheter-related infection is minimized. Other veins in the neck can be used. The common facial vein is very useful in infants.

The internal jugular vein can be used directly. This vein should not be ligated. Place a purse-string suture of 5-0 cardiovascular Prolene in the vein. Make a stab wound in the center of the purse-string and place the catheter in the vein.

The saphenous vein in the ankle is a large constant vein that can be used in an emergency. It is easy to locate (Fig. 7-20), even

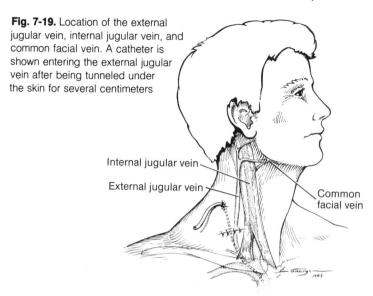

Fig. 7-19. Location of the external jugular vein, internal jugular vein, and common facial vein. A catheter is shown entering the external jugular vein after being tunneled under the skin for several centimeters

Internal jugular vein

External jugular vein

Common facial vein

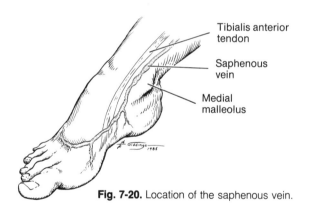

Tibialis anterior tendon

Saphenous vein

Medial malleolus

Fig. 7-20. Location of the saphenous vein.

when collapsed. Make a transverse incision from the tibialis anterior tendon to the medial malleolus. Pass a curved clamp from the medial malleolus, deep along the fibrous capsule of the ankle joint, and emerging next to the tibialis anterior tendon. The vein will be contained in the tissue isolated by the clamp. Dissect with a second clamp to locate the vein.

Technique of cutdown

Begin any cutdown by locating the vein. Except for the cephalic vein, it should be possible to identify the vein beneath the skin. This makes it possible to use a very small incision and avoids a long and frustrating dissection.

Prepare the skin and drape the field. Make a small (1 to 2 cm) incision transversely over the vein. Spread gently with a curved clamp until the vein is reached. Clear the vein for 1 or 2 cm. Pass ties, (2-0 or 3-0 silk) around the vein proximally and distally. Tie distally (Fig. 7-21). Pick up the vein 2 or 3 mm from the distal tie

Fig. 7-21. Venous cutdown technique.

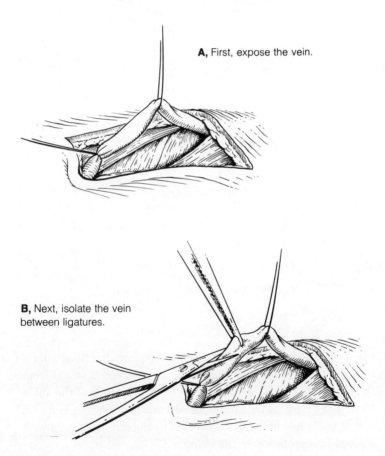

A, First, expose the vein.

B, Next, isolate the vein between ligatures.

Fig. 7-21, cont'd. Venous cutdown technique.

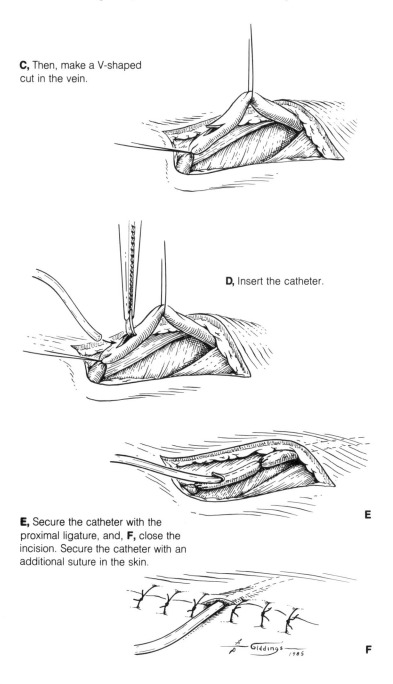

C, Then, make a V-shaped
cut in the vein.

D, Insert the catheter.

E, Secure the catheter with the
proximal ligature, and, **F,** close the
incision. Secure the catheter with an
additional suture in the skin.

E

F

Fig. 7-22. Alternate technique of venous cutdown.

A and **B,** The catheter enters the skin and,

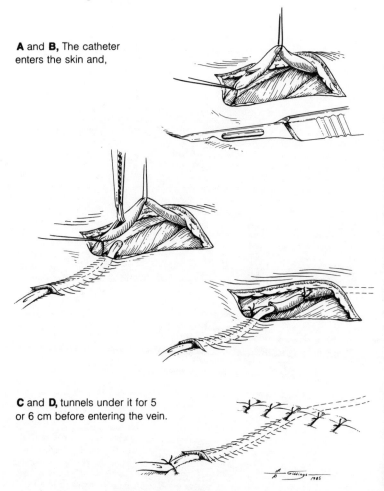

C and **D,** tunnels under it for 5 or 6 cm before entering the vein.

This technique helps avoid phlebitis in long-term catheterization.

with a fine forceps. Cut the vein with fine-pointed scissors using a V-shaped cut. Pick up the apex of the V-shaped flap with the forceps; this spreads the vein open and helps with insertion of the catheter. Now insert the catheter. This is easier said than done because the vein collapses and usually goes into spasm. The catheter, which should be a little smaller than the distended vein, looks larger than the collapsed vessel. It is helpful to have a

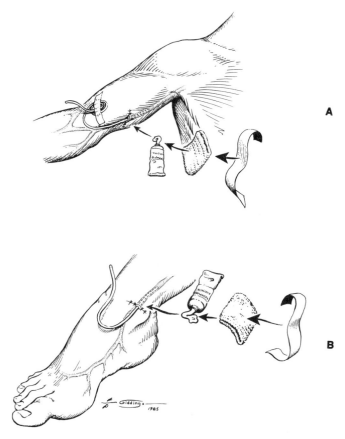

Fig. 7-23. Dressing techniques for venous catheters. **A,** Brachial catheter. **B,** Saphenous catheter.

bevel on the catheter. When the bevel is cut, be sure to blunt the point to avoid damage to the vein. After putting the catheter in the vein, thread it to the desired position, and tie the proximal ligature around both the vein and catheter. Suture the wound by bringing the catheter out through the wound or through a separate stab wound (Fig. 7-22). As the catheter emerges from the skin, place a suture in the skin and wrap it two or three times around the catheter to further secure it. Loop the catheter back on itself and secure it in a manner similar to other venous cannulus (Fig. 7-23). Cover the wound and exit site with iodophor ointment and a sterile occlusive dressing.

PULMONARY ARTERY CATHETER

The thermistor-tipped pulmonary artery catheter is best known as the Swan-Ganz catheter, but a number of manufacturers make identical catheters. These are designed for placement in the pulmonary artery for measurement of the pulmonary capillary wedge pressure (PCWP) and the cardiac output (Fig. 7-24). A pulmonary artery catheter is used to estimate left ventricular filling pressure because the central venous pressure is a poor index of the state of the circulation. If the left atrial pressure, the arterial pressure, and the cardiac output are known, the state of the left ventricle can be assessed precisely. In addition, pulmonary edema can be avoided by monitoring the left atrial pressure. However, the left atrium is inaccessible. When a catheter is placed into the pulmonary artery and then wedged into a pulmonary artery branch, the resultant pulmonary capillary wedge pressure (PCWP) reflects the left atrial pressure reasonably well (Fig. 7-25).

Using a catheter with the tip in the pulmonary artery allows determination of the cardiac output. A thermistor is located in the catheter just proximal to the balloon (Fig. 7-24). Cool saline is injected into the right atrium through a separate lumen. Mixing takes place in the right ventricle. The temperature curve traced by the thermistor is used to calculate the cardiac output. There are microprocessor-based devices available that will measure the temperature of the injected saline, monitor the thermistor, perform the calculations, and indicate the cardiac output on a digital readout on the front panel.

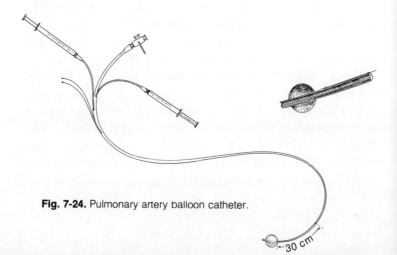

Fig. 7-24. Pulmonary artery balloon catheter.

Several techniques can be employed to place a pulmonary artery catheter. A brachial cutdown can be used. The most common technique is the infraclavicular puncture incorporating an over-needle catheter. The major difficulty is passing the balloon-tipped catheter through the right side of the heart.

The technique of passing the catheter is the same as for central venous catheterization (p. 112). Thread the catheter into the right atrium, then connect the distal lumen to a pressure gauge. The pressure tracing should be a right atrial (RA) pressure (Fig. 7-26). Inflate the balloon. The inflated balloon "floats" the tip

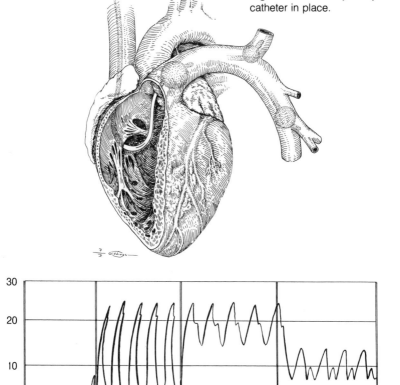

Fig. 7-25. Pulmonary artery catheter in place.

Fig. 7-26. Pressures obtained as the pulmonary artery catheter is advanced into the right atrium *(RA)*, the right ventricle *(RV)*, the pulmonary artery *(PA)*, and the wedge position *(PCW)*.

into the right ventricle (RV) and pulmonary artery (PA). Advance the catheter gently. As the tip enters the right ventricle, the ventricular pressure tracing, shown in Fig. 7-26, should appear. Continue to advance the catheter until a pulmonary artery tracing is seen. Advance a little further into the wedge position. It may be necessary to deflate the balloon, advance 2 or 3 cm, and reinflate the balloon. The tracing should show a much lower pressure, which should have an atrial form, as shown in the figure. The RA pressure and the PCW pressure show two elevations per cardiac cycle, whereas the RV and PA pressures show only one. Connect the pressure gauge to the proximal lumen; this should show a right atrial pressure. If it shows a right ventricular pressure, the catheter is too far in and should be pulled back. The injection opening should be in the right atrium and the tip in the pulmonary artery. Lastly, suture the skin, secure the catheter, and dress as for any other cutdown catheter. Be especially careful to secure the catheter to the skin; it is vital that the catheter not be moved.

The pulmonary artery catheter is indicated in only a few situations. One major indication is the necessity for pharmacologic support of the circulation (pressors, vasodilators) in a patient who has clinical signs of cardiovascular compromise. This includes cardiogenic shock, septic shock, severe electrolyte abnormalities, severe burns, and postoperative cardiovascular instability. It is not desirable to leave a pulmonary artery catheter in place longer than 72 hours. It often stops working. The PCW pressure becomes less accurate, presumably because of thrombosis of the artery distal to the catheter. There is also a risk of thrombosis and emboli. The catheter traverses the right ventricular outflow tract, which is notoriously sensitive to mechanical stimuli, and may cause arrhythmias. For all of these reasons the catheter should be removed as soon as the patient's condition is reasonably stable.

8

Arterial techniques

The need for access to the arterial circulation is not as common as for venous cannulation. However, in critically ill patients it is often necessary to monitor the blood pressure or determine blood gases. In some radiologic procedures access to an artery is necessary.

ARTERIAL PUNCTURE

The usual reason for arterial puncture is to obtain arterial blood for pH, P_{O_2}, and P_{CO_2}. The easiest artery to puncture is the radial artery at the wrist, although the femoral artery in the groin and the brachial artery at the elbow are sometimes used.

The familiar radial pulse is medial to the radial styloid, where the radial artery goes over the lower end of the radius (Fig. 8-1). To puncture the artery, use a short, fine needle (25 gauge, 5/8 inch) on the syringe to be used for the sample, usually a 2.5 or 5 ml syringe with one or two drops of heparin solution. Prepare the skin with iodophor. Introduce the needle perpendicular to the skin over the artery, about 1 cm proximal to the tip of the radial styloid. Puncture the skin, carefully locate the artery, and impale the artery with the needle. Arteries are hard to puncture. An artery is thick-walled, smaller, and more likely than a vein to move out of the way of the needle. The best technique is to push the needle firmly into the artery without worrying about going through the other side. If the needle is in too far (Fig. 8-1, C), it should be pulled back far enough to allow a free flow of blood into the syringe. After removing the needle, keep pressure on the site for 5 to 10 minutes.

The two major advantages of the radial artery are its superficial location and its lack of an accompanying vein. Any blood obtained is going to be arterial blood. All other accessible arteries are accompanied by veins.

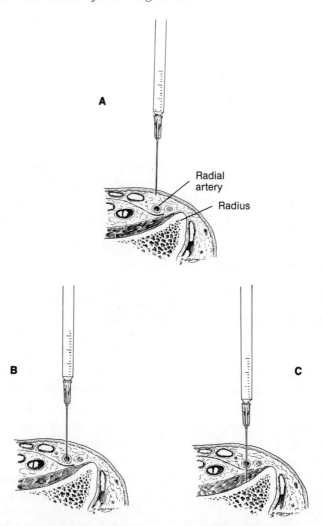

Fig. 8-1. Arterial puncture of the radial artery at the wrist. **A,** The needle has entered the skin. **B,** The needle is in the artery in good position. **C,** The needle has impaled the artery and must be pulled back.

The other commonly used arteries are the brachial and the femoral. In both cases it is necessary to distinguish between an arterial and venous puncture. If the blood is red and pushes the plunger of the syringe back, there is no question that it is an arterial puncture. However, if the patient has hypoxemia, the arterial blood may be dark.

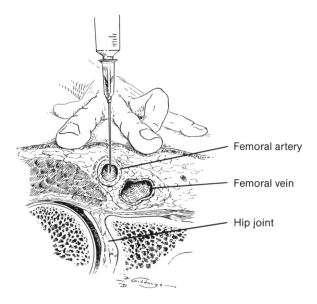

Fig. 8-2. Technique of femoral artery puncture.

With the elbow fully extended, locate the brachial artery about 1 cm above the elbow crease. Prepare the skin with iodophor. Using a short, 25-gauge needle, puncture the skin perpendicularly and impale the artery. Withdraw the needle until blood is obtained. Verify that the blood is arterial. Keep pressure on the artery for 10 minutes after drawing the sample to control bleeding.

Femoral puncture is useful for sampling when the arm vessels cannot be used. A 25-gauge, 5/8 inch needle is sometimes adequate, especially in a thin patient, but a 22-gauge, 1 or 1 1/2 inch needle is usually better. The artery is fairly easy to locate. Place a finger on either side of the artery and puncture the skin perpendicularly (Fig. 8-2). Impale the artery, draw back until the tip is in the artery, and obtain the sample. Be sure the sample is arterial. The femoral artery is fairly large but is also fairly mobile, therefore it is much easier to puncture the less mobile and larger femoral vein.

ARTERIAL CANNULATION

The availability of the over-needle cannulas has made it possible to cannulate arteries percutaneously (Fig. 8-3). These cannulas are available in 20 gauge, 1 1/2 inch size for this purpose. The technique is very much the same as for venous cannulation. Prepare the skin with iodophor. Puncture the skin with the needle, then puncture the artery. Advance a little farther along the artery to ensure that the cannula enters the artery, and finally slide the cannula over the needle. Pull the needle out and place a three-way stopcock on the cannula. It is best to use a stopcock with Luer-Lok fittings so that the stopcock cannot come loose; patients have bled to death through a disconnected arterial cannula. The radial artery is used almost exclusively for this purpose. Theoretically, a cannula can be left in place for several days and then pulled out without thrombosing the artery. In practice, the artery usually remains occluded. The danger of thrombosis makes it a little risky to cannulate the brachial or femoral arteries, although either is safe for short periods.

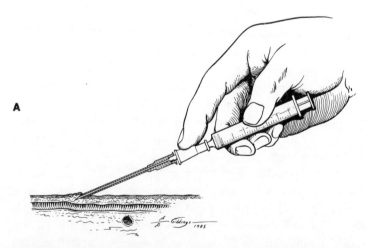

A

Fig. 8-3. Cannulation of an artery with an over-needle cannula. In **A,** the needle and catheter have been inserted through the skin. In **B,** the needle tip has been inserted into the vein. Blood can be aspirated, but the catheter is not yet in the artery. **C,** Raise the needle tip and advance the needle further so that the catheter enters the artery. **D,** Thread the catheter over the needle, into the artery, and remove the needle.

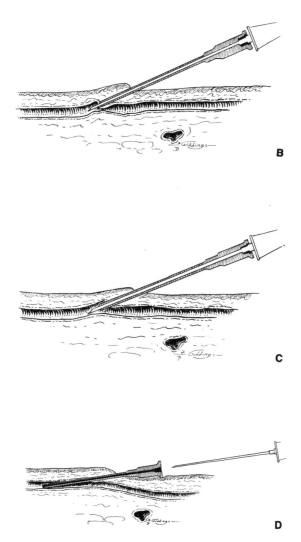

Fig. 8-3, cont'd. For legend see opposite page.

ARTERIAL CUTDOWN

Arterial cutdown formerly was the only available method for cannulating an artery for monitoring purposes. With the use of arterial cannulation by over-needle cannulas and the availability of the Doppler flow detector for obtaining blood pressures, arterial cutdowns are less common. However, they are still necessary in children and occasionally in adults.

The technique almost always demands the radial artery. No other artery is as large and accessible and yet can be tied off without harm. In neonates, the umbilical artery may be cannulated by dissecting through the upper midline of the abdomen into the ligamentum teres.

The factor that makes the radial artery safe is that the hand is adequately supplied by both the radial and ulnar arteries, which connect through the deep and superficial palmar arches (Fig. 8-4). To verify that the radial artery can be ligated, perform the

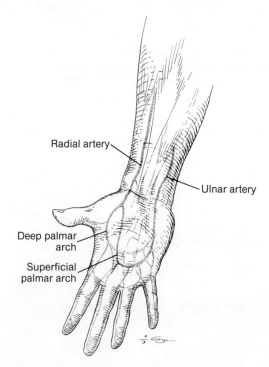

Fig. 8-4. Anatomy of the radial and ulnar arteries and the superficial and deep palmar arches.

Allen test (Fig. 8-5). Using both hands, compress the radial and ulnar arteries at the wrist. Raise the patient's hand over his head and have him clench his fist several times. This should result in a pale, cool hand. Let the patient relax his hand. Take the pressure off the ulnar artery. The hand should become pink immediately. If it stays pale but becomes pink when the radial artery is released, a radial cutdown is not safe. A Doppler flow detector can also be used to determine ulnar artery patency.

The technique for arterial cutdown is the same as for venous cutdown (Fig. 8-6). A shorter, finer cannula can be used. Special care should be taken to use a catheter with a molded hub; a No. 18 or No. 20 over-needle cannula is ideal. The hub should be connected to a three-way, Luer-Lok stopcock.

One modification of the arterial cutdown technique should be considered (Fig. 8-7). In this modification the artery is isolated and controlled with a ligature. An over-needle cannula is then inserted through the skin distal to the incision. The cannula is

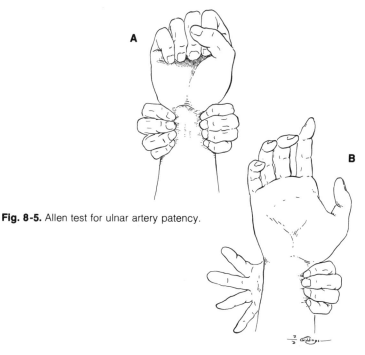

Fig. 8-5. Allen test for ulnar artery patency.

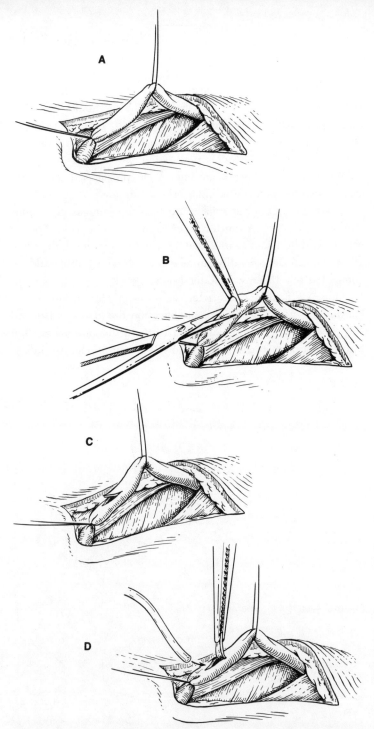

Fig. 8-6. Open cannulation of the radial artery, using cutdown technique.

E

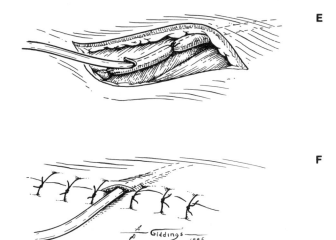

F

Fig. 8-6, cont'd. For legend see opposite page.

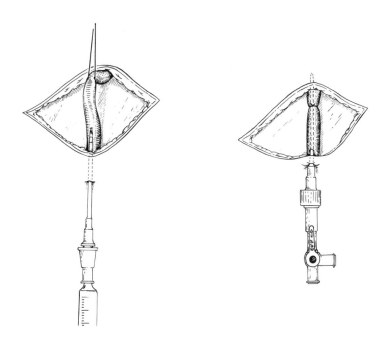

Fig. 8-7. Open cannulation of radial artery using an over-needle cannula.

inserted into the artery under direct vision. Absorbable suture material is then used to ligate the artery around the cannula. The distal artery is not ligated. In theory this allows preservation of the artery, but in practice the artery usually thromboses.

Care of the arterial line is somewhat more demanding than the venous line. Irrigation must be frequent, to avoid clotting, but must be carefully done. Irrigation of as little as 2 ml of saline can cause reflux of clots up the carotid artery. All particulate matter and especially all clots must be removed by aspiration. No air bubbles should be allowed in the system. Heparinized saline must be used for all irrigations. Devices are available that will continuously and slowly infuse heparinized saline into the line; these are helpful, but frequent monitoring and periodic irrigation are still necessary.

9

Biopsy techniques

Much of diagnostic medicine consists of techniques for obtaining tissue for microscopic analysis. Although some of these techniques are so complicated that entire specialties have been built around them, others should be part of the repertoire of any physician. These include open biopsy of the skin and subcutaneous tissues, punch biopsy, needle biopsy, and liver biopsy.

The basic purpose of performing a biopsy is to obtain a diagnosis. Obviously, tissue should be sent to the pathologist. But the diagnosis may be obtained in the bacteriology lab. All specimens should be cultured for aerobic and anaerobic bacteria, mycobacteria, and fungi.

INCISIONAL BIOPSY

Incisional biopsy is shown for skin lesions (Fig. 9-1) and for deep lesions (Fig. 9-2). For both, begin by preparing a wide area of skin and placing drapes. Use infiltration anesthesia or regional block. If a small electrocautery is available, it can be used to control bleeding vessels in the subcutaneous tissues.

For small skin lesions, the basic technique is to make the incision as a pointed oval in Langer's lines (Fig. 5-1), staying 2 or 3 mm from the lesion. Take the whole lesion as well as a wedge of subcutaneous tissue. This ensures that the deep margin of the lesion is removed and makes the closure somewhat easier. For any incision longer than 1 or 2 cm, a few deep sutures of absorbable suture should be placed below the skin to close dead space and help approximate the skin. Suture the skin with fine nonabsorbable suture, such as 4-0 nylon. The technique is the same as for suturing lacerations, described in Chapter 6.

For deeper lesions, the first rule is to make absolutely sure that the lesion can be located. Many lesions, especially those deep in areas such as the axilla or the breast, can be palpated only

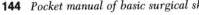

Fig. 9-1. Basic technique for skin lesions.

Fig. 9-2. Basic technique for deep lesions.

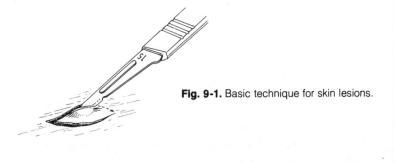

in certain positions. It is frustrating to prepare the skin, drape the field, infiltrate the skin with local anesthetic, and then realize that the lesion can no longer be felt. It is extremely important to place the incision exactly over the nodule. If the incision is even 1 or 2 cm from a small nodule, it can be very difficult to locate the nodule and carry out a clean biopsy. Once the nodule is located, place the incision in Langer's lines. Dissect down to the nodule. Grasp the tissue immediately surrounding the nodule or the area involved, hold it up, and dissect around the nodule with a knife or scissors until it is free. This inevitably leaves several bleeding vessels in the deep portion of the wound. Clamp them and either cauterize them with the electrocautery or tie them with fine suture. In the subcutaneous nodule it is especially important to close the subcutaneous tissue and eliminate dead space. This prevents the formation of a hematoma or seroma and aids in closure of the skin.

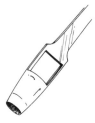

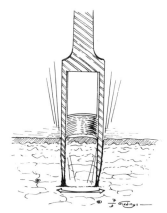

Fig. 9-3. Use of punch biopsy instrument.

It is important to know when not to do a biopsy. A nodule in the neck is the most usual situation in which a biopsy should be avoided. The presence of a neck mass should lead to a diagnostic evaluation aimed at detecting a cancer in the head or neck, including careful laryngoscopy, pharyngoscopy, meticulous examination of the mouth and tongue, examination of the nasopharynx, and x-ray films of the sinuses. Only after a detailed examination is completely negative should a biopsy be performed on a suspicious nodule in the neck.

There are a number of modifications of the incisional biopsy technique for special purposes. For example, in diagnosing certain types of muscular diseases it is necessary to obtain a piece of muscle. Generally, the gastrocnemius muscle in the calf is used. A small transverse incision is placed in the upper portion of the calf. A portion of the muscle is dissected free, isolated between ligatures, and excised. It is often desirable to include a small nerve with the specimen, especially in the analysis of neuromuscular disorders.

PUNCH BIOPSY

Punch biopsy is a useful technique in the diagnosis of large or fungating skin lesions. The biopsy punch looks like a modified cork borer (Fig. 9-3). It is available in sizes ranging from 2 to 6 mm in diameter. The most useful size is 3 mm.

Prepare the skin well. Drape towels are not necessary and the procedure requires gloves only. Infiltrate the involved area. Perform the biopsy by placing the open mouth of the punch on the lesion and pressing down while rotating the punch. This "cores out" a piece of tissue the diameter of the punch. The piece of tissue is still attached on its deep margin and can be detached in a number of ways: (1) move the punch from side to side, scraping the lesion from the underlying tissue, (2) angulate the punch one way and then another way, cutting the deep margin with the edge of the punch, or (3) remove the punch, pick up the lesion with the forceps, and divide its base with iris scissors. Close the hole with a single suture, if necessary, to stop any bleeding.

It is important to know where to perform the biopsy. Because the punch biopsy provides a relatively small tissue sample, it should be obtained as close to the margin of the lesion as possible. This provides considerably more information than performing a biopsy at the center. In large lesions the center is often necrotic, infected, or ulcerated, and is difficult to examine under the microscope. The edge of the lesion near normal tissue is usually the most representative portion. If a specimen can be obtained precisely at the area at which the lesion joins normal tissue, so much the better. But if it is important to do the biopsy at the exact margin, incisional biopsy is a better technique.

NEEDLE BIOPSY

The most commonly used biopsy needle—the Tru-Cut, by Travenol is shown here (Fig. 9-4). Its use is simple. Advance the needle until it just enters the lesion. Push the inner portion of the needle into the lesion. Then advance the outer needle over the inner portion and pull out both parts of the needle together. The resulting core of tissue is 2 cm long and 1 mm in diameter.

LIVER BIOPSY

Of all the major organs, the liver is most commonly biopsied. Biopsy is indicated in diseases such as cirrhosis of the liver, but it is also useful in diagnosing metastatic cancer. Do not perform a biopsy on patients whose prothrombin time is prolonged or who have ascites. In either case the liver wound may not stop bleeding.

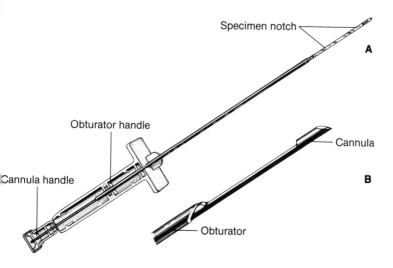

Fig. 9-4. Biopsy needle, Tru-cut. **A,** Biopsy needle. **B,** Detail of the specimen notch.

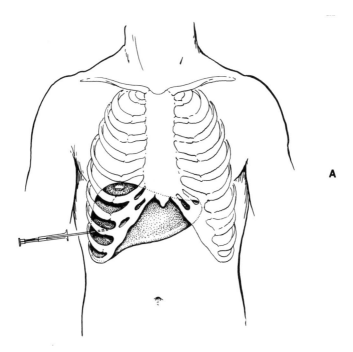

Fig. 9-5. Technique for liver biopsy. **A,** Site of biopsy.
Continued.

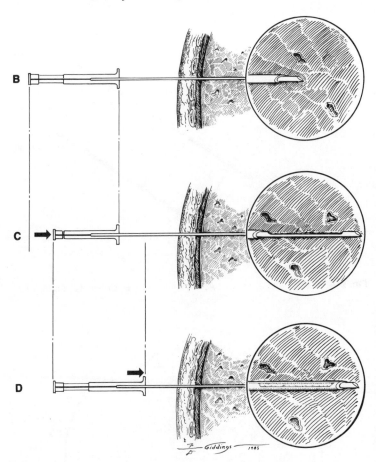

Fig. 9-5, cont'd. B, Insert needle. **C,** Advance inner part of needle into liver. **D,** Advance outer part of needle, cutting off biopsy.

Prepare and drape the skin over the liver. The liver generally does not come down to the costal margin, but it descends with inspiration. If the needle is inserted between the anterior and midaxillary lines in the eighth or ninth intercostal space and advanced at right angles to the skin, the right lateral lobe of the liver will be perforated. This approach is unlikely to result in injury to the gallbladder or to the hepatic ducts. The entire maneuver should be done while the patient is holding his breath, because the liver moves with breathing. It is helpful to have the patient hold his breath at inspiration, so the liver will be relatively far down. Advance the needle approximately 3 to 4 cm through the chest wall and the attachments of the diaphragm. The needle can usually be felt to enter the liver. Advance the inner portion to its full length, then push the outer portion over it (Fig. 9-5). Remove the needle. The whole technique should take 5 to 10 seconds.

If an adequate piece of tissue is obtained at the first biopsy, the procedure should be terminated. Often it takes two or three biopsies before enough tissue is obtained. When the procedure is unsuccessful after three attempts at needle biopsy, it should be terminated. Failure after an adequate effort generally means that there is some other factor involved. Either the liver is too small and not in the normal position, or it is too hard and cirrhotic. Persistence in this particular situation is not a virtue. It may produce damage and rarely produces a diagnosis.

10

Drainage of body cavities

One of the major medical advances of the past 50 years has been virtually unlimited access to the major body cavities. This has been made possible both by the use of aseptic technique and by the availability of suitable needles and cannulas. In its way, access to the body cavities has been as dramatic a development as the use of intravenous techniques. It has allowed aspiration for diagnostic purposes and drainage for therapy. Practically all body cavities are now accessible to the probing needle. Some areas, such as the ventricles of the brain and the capsules of joints, are of interest largely to specialists. The areas most physicians routinely deal with are the pleural cavity, pericardial cavity, peritoneal cavity, and the subarachnoid space.

PLEURAL CAVITY

Drainage of the pleural cavity is common. The basic technique is thoracentesis (Fig. 10-1). The exact site of thoracentesis depends on the location of the fluid within the chest. Most commonly the fluid is basal and posterior. The best location for thoracentesis is between the posterior axillary line and the midscapular line, in the eighth or ninth intercostal space. A relatively long, large-bore needle should be used. The bevel should be as short as feasible to minimize the chance of lacerating the lung. Forty-five degree bevel needles are commonly used, in contrast with the much longer bevel needles used for venipuncture.

Put the patient in a sitting position. If possible, the best position is sitting backward in a chair and resting the arms and shoulders on the back of the chair. Prepare the skin of the back. The upright position makes it difficult to drape the patient. Usually it is sufficient to place a single towel immediately below the thoracentesis site. Raise a skin wheal by injecting local anesthetic at the proposed site. Place the large needle through this skin

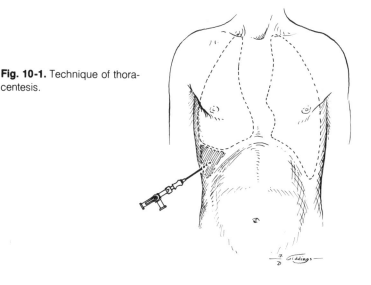

Fig. 10-1. Technique of thora-centesis.

wheal. It is best to puncture the skin first with a No. 11 blade and to introduce the needle through the small stab wound. Pass the needle through the intercostal space immediately over a rib. The intercostal bundle is located at the lower edge of the rib. The pleura can usually be felt as a resistance to the passage of the needle; the needle will "pop" through the pleura. Push the needle into the pleural space a very short distance and then aspirate. If a free flow of fluid is obtained, keep the needle at that position by clamping across the needle flush with the skin. Using the three-way stopcock and a large syringe, remove fluid. For diagnosis only, aspirate 20 cc of fluid. But most often a thera-peutic thoracentesis is done. In this case take out as much fluid as possible. However, be aware that removal of more than 1000 cc may disturb the patient's fluid balance and may cause hypoten-sion. Once the fluid has been removed, withdraw the needle and place a Band-Aid over the puncture site. A chest x-ray examina-tion is indicated upon completion of thoracentesis.

The most dangerous part of the thoracentesis is at the end. As the last of the fluid is withdrawn, the lung comes up to the chest wall. If the needle protrudes too far into the pleural space, it may lacerate the lung. One way of avoiding this is to use a flexible catheter, usually an over-needle or through-needle catheter.

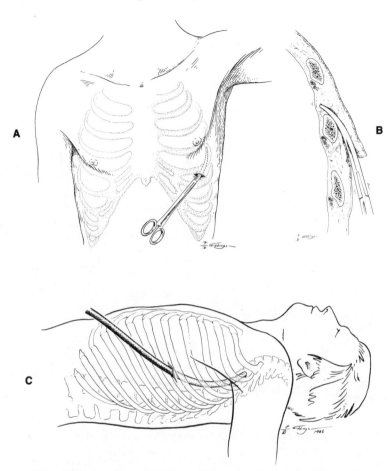

Fig. 10-2. Placing a chest tube. **A,** Site. **B,** Dissecting through chest wall. **C,** Final position.

Once a catheter has been placed into the pleural space, fluid can be aspirated from it without fear that the lung will be lacerated by the soft plastic. This technique is especially good for removing a large volume of fluid.

Placement of a chest tube is often necessary for the removal of fluid, evacuation of hemopneumothorax, or pneumothorax (Fig. 10-2). The best site is between the anterior and midaxillary line in the seventh, eighth, or ninth interspaces (Fig. 10-2, *A*). Occasionally a patient will require an anterior chest tube, which is usually placed through the first or second intercostal space in the midclavicular line. The use of a high axillary tube should be avoided because this type of tube is painful and interferes with motion of the arm. The tube passes through an area containing sweat glands and is therefore vulnerable to infection.

Place the patient on his side, prepare and drape a wide area. Anesthetize the skin over the proposed site. It is very helpful to place a rib block 3 or 4 inches posterior to the desired site and blocking four or five interspaces. Make a 2 cm skin incision on top of a rib. Dissect obliquely backward along and over the rib into the interspace (Fig. 10-2, *B*). Push the clamp through the pleura. Penetration of the pleura usually produces sharp pain, although this can be prevented by a rib block. Enlarge the opening and place a larger clamp beside the small clamp used for the dissection. Pass the tube between the jaws of the larger clamp and direct it into the pleural space. The tube should spiral up into the apex of the chest. A stylet is helpful in placing a 28 French (or smaller) tube.

For empyema the technique is a little different. The object is to place the tube directly through the chest wall into the cavity. Locate the cavity with x-ray films or ultrasound and mark the chest wall. Using a rib block, explore with a needle to verify that the cavity is located. Make a 2 to 3 cm incision over the interspace and bluntly dissect straight through into the chest. Placing a finger in the chest, explore the cavity and break up any loculations. Then insert a 36 French (or larger) tube directly in the space.

Secure the tube with a simple suture of heavy braided polyester or silk (Fig. 10-3). Tie it with the first throw of a surgeon's knot, but not so tightly as to necrose the skin. Wrap the suture around the tube many times and tie. When removing the tube, cut the knot and unwind the suture. Enough length will be left to tie the suture after removal of the chest tube (Fig. 10-4). Connect the chest tube to underwater seal drainage and apply a dressing around the tube. The pleural space tends to protect itself against infection quite well, and antibiotic coverage of a patient with a chest tube is not necessary. However, it is best to protect the skin opening with a dressing.

Management of a chest tube requires an understanding of exactly what happens in the pleural space. The pleural space normally contains no air and a very small amount of fluid. Because of the elastic recoil of the lungs, the intrapleural pressure is

Fig. 10-3. Securing a chest tube—
single suture technique. The suture
should be loose, and the surgeon's
knot tied down loosely. A tight suture
may cause skin necrosis.

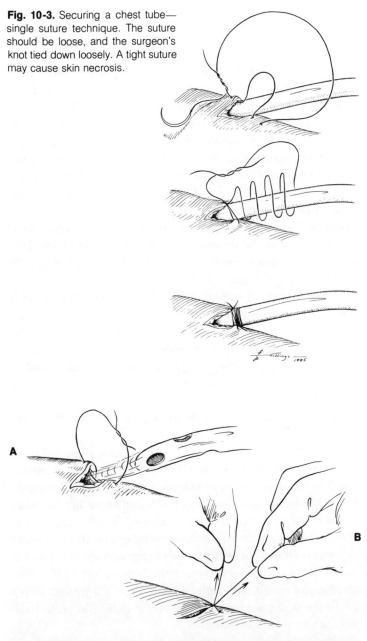

Fig. 10-4. Removing a chest tube. The single suture technique can be used
(Fig. 10-3). **A,** Unwrap the suture from around the tube. Have the patient
breathe in and then do a Valsalva maneuver. Pull the tube. **B,** Tie the suture
down while the patient is still straining down.

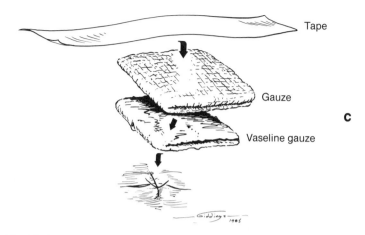

Tape

Gauze

Vaseline gauze

C

Fig. 10-4, cont'd. C, Place Vaseline gauze over the wound, to further occlude the tract, and cover this with gauze and tape.

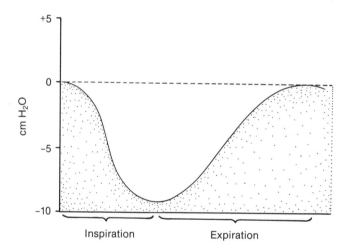

cm H_2O

+5

0

-5

-10

Inspiration

Expiration

Fig. 10-5. Pressure in the pleural space.

negative. It changes with respiration, as shown in Fig. 10-5. During expiration it rises to zero, but during normal inspiration it falls to around -10 cm of water. Because of this negative pressure, an open tube placed in the pleural space would allow air to rush in and collapse the lung. So it is necessary to connect a valve to the end of the tube. This valve will allow fluid and air to leave the pleural space but will not allow air to come back in.

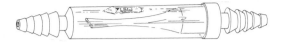

Fig. 10-6. Heimlich valve.

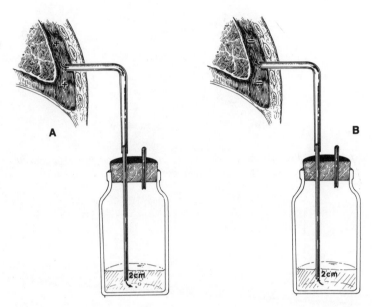

Fig. 10-7. Chest tube and chest bottle. **A,** Air escaping on expiration, with positive pleural pressure. **B,** Air unable to enter on inspiration, with negative pressure.

The simplest form of valve is the Heimlich valve (Fig. 10-6). This valve is simple, easy to understand, and portable. It is especially useful for transporting patients with chest tubes. However, it has two major disadvantages. First, it offers resistance to air leaving the pleural space. Second, in the presence of protein-containing fluid, the valve may stick shut and stop working.

The most commonly used one-way valve is the chest bottle (Fig. 10-7). The chest tube is connected to a glass or plastic tube, the end of which is under 1 to 2 cm of water. This allows air to bubble out relatively freely but prevents air or fluid from coming back into the chest. A pneumothorax can be expanded with a chest bottle alone. If, with each breath, 10 to 20 ml of air bubbles out and none bubbles back in, the pneumothorax will be evacu-

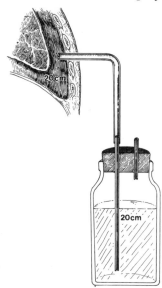

Fig. 10-8. Full chest bottle, showing that there is a 20 cm of back pressure on the one-way valve.

ated in a few minutes. Similarly, fluid will drain out the tube and into the bottle and not reenter the chest.

As the bottle fills up, it offers resistance to flow (Fig. 10-8). If the bottle has 20 cm of fluid in it, then 20 cm of pressure is required to force air out of the chest. This prevents air and fluid from leaving the chest. Accordingly suction is commonly used.

Suction is perhaps the most misunderstood aspect of chest tube management. The mechanism of producing suction is somewhat confusing and the indications for its use are still more so.

A low suction in the range of −10 to −40 cm of water is required. If more than −40 cm of water pressure is applied to a tube in the pleural space, pain is produced. Even smaller amounts of suction can sometimes be painful. The lung is pulled up against the chest wall by the tube, stimulating pain receptors in both the parietal and visceral pleura. So relatively low suction, usually −20 cm of water (−15 mm Hg), is required. But in the event an air leak is present, a relatively large flow may be required. Peak flow (on coughing) may be as high as 50 L/min.

Perhaps the simplest and best device for producing suction is the fan-operated Emerson suction machine. The fan is inherently a high-flow, low-suction device. The speed of the fan is controlled by a rheostat, and the pressure is read from a meter on the front panel. When the unit is off, the chest bottle is open to the air between the fan blades, so that the device is safe even if accidentally turned off. The fan can remove a large volume of air at a constant pressure, so that even the largest air leak can be managed. Several companies (Ohmeda, Puritan-Bennett) make wall-mounted regulators for chest suction. Most regulators for gastric or endotracheal suction operate in the range of 80 to 200 mm Hg. The chest suction regulators work from 0 to 60 mm Hg (0 to 80 cm water). These regulators have high flow capacity and are very convenient to use.

Often a modification of the old three-bottle system (Fig. 10-9) is used to produce suction. The full-fledged three-bottle system consists of three separate units—a trap bottle, a chest bottle, and a vacuum regulator bottle. The trap bottle can fill without changing the pressure relationships of the system, and it prevents the chest bottle from filling. The vacuum regulator bottle is connected to wall suction and is filled to about 20 cm. The long tube is open to the atmosphere and the tip extends 20 cm below the surface of the water. One of the short tubes is connected to the chest bottle and the other is connected to wall suction. The wall

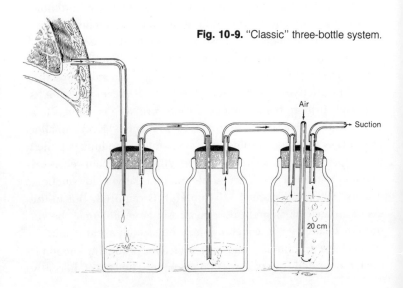

Fig. 10-9. "Classic" three-bottle system.

Air

Suction

20 cm

suction, at 500 to 600 mm Hg, is far in excess of what is needed. As wall suction is applied to the bottle, it reaches a value of −20 cm rather quickly. At this value air is pulled in through the long tube. This limits the pressure in the bottle to −20 cm. To prevent the flow of air through the bottle from becoming too vigorous, the needle valve on the wall suction regulator is turned down to permit only a relatively small flow of air through the device. Unfortunately, this limits the capacity of the system to extract air from the patient. This in turn is the same as the amount of air that is pulled through the long tube and allowed to bubble through the suction regulator bottle. If this capacity is exceeded, the system can become dangerous. A patient with a large air leak not only can cut off the flow of air through the system but can generate a positive air pressure in the system. A patient, on coughing, may actually force water out of the upper end of the long tube. Nonetheless, this system (or modifications of it) is very useful for managing the patient whose suction requirements are not critical. This includes patients with copious fluid drainage, postoperative cardiac patients, or patients needing suction and having no air leak.

The commercially available versions of this system are one-piece disposable plastic units containing all three chambers—collection chamber, chest bottle chamber, and suction chamber—in a molded configuration. They are connected to the patient and to wall suction. These disposable units are convenient to use but expensive (Figs. 10-10, *A* and 10-10, *B*).

The major disadvantages of the bubbler systems are their relative complexity and low flow capacity. It is very common to see the commercial units connected erroneously, even on an intensive care unit. The simple chest bottle, in conjunction with the fan suction device or a wall-mounted regulator, is easier to teach people to use. But all forms of chest suction devices are prone to errors in technique that stem from ignorance of the basic principles of the system.

The question of when to use suction is always puzzling because the decision is frequently arbitrary. The most common reason for using suction was mentioned earlier. When a chest bottle fills up, it produces back pressure in the thorax (Fig. 10-8). To overcome 20 cm of back pressure, simply put −20 cm of

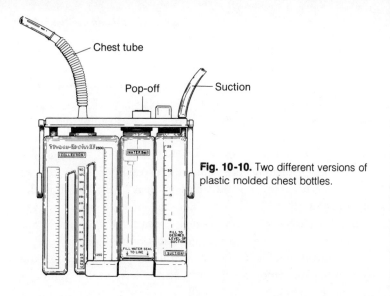

Chest tube

Pop-off

Suction

Fig. 10-10. Two different versions of plastic molded chest bottles.

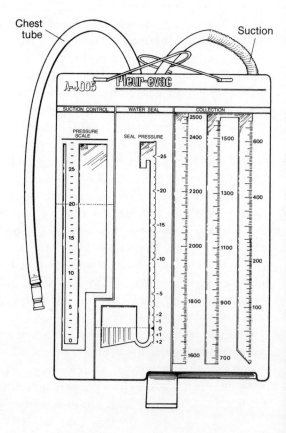

Chest tube

Suction

suction on the bottle. In some situations the use of suction is important for other reasons. The first such situation is the presence of a large air leak. A simple chest tube and chest bottle system may not remove air fast enough. A suction system of some sort is required to get the air out of the chest fast enough to keep ahead of the leak and expand the lung. When the lung expands, it comes into contact with the visceral pleura; and it is apparently this contact that seals leaks from the lung. A large air leak is most common postoperatively. It is also seen in some cases of spontaneous pneumothorax and in trauma. A second situation in which suction is almost universally used is following trauma. The object is to evacuate the blood in the chest as fast as possible, to prevent it from clotting, to expand the lung, and to tamponade the bleeding vessels. There is very often an associated air leak. A third situation requiring suction involves the postoperative cardiac patient. Generally, mediastinal tubes are used. Although the pleural cavity may be opened during the operation, normally it is not. Mediastinal tubes act like wound suction catheters. There is rarely an air leak, and the major purpose of the tube is to remove fluid. Suction is almost universally used.

The major indication for removing the chest tube is that it has done its job. It is relatively unimportant whether or not the tube is fluctuating. The tube fluctuates as long as it communicates with the free pleural space. After the tube has been in place for a week or so, the parietal pleura tends to seal to the visceral pleura around the tube, thus excluding the tube from the free pleural space. At this point the tube stops fluctuating. It can, in fact, be cut off and the lung will not collapse. The lung is now held to the chest wall by adhesions. In spontaneous pneumothorax the tube should be removed as soon as the lung is expanded and the air leak has stopped. If there has been a prolonged air leak, it is good to keep the tube in for 48 hours after the last air leak. In either case the tube can be fluctuating when it is removed. On the other hand, in empyema, even though the tube has stopped fluctuating, it is usually too early to remove it. The empyema tube functions as a drain in an abscess cavity. If it is removed too quickly, the abscess will recur. In using an empyema tube, the classic technique is to cut the tube off at the chest wall, allow it to drain into a dressing, and remove it at the rate of 2 inches per week for several weeks.

When removing a chest tube, it is very important, especially if the tube is fluctuating, to block passage of air back into the pleural space. The best way of doing this is to use a suture at the tube entry site (Figs. 10-3 and 10-4). The suture can be placed either at the time of initial tube placement (Fig. 10-3) or at removal. A second way of sealing the opening is with Vaseline gauze, which supposedly makes an airtight seal. However, the Vaseline may interfere with taping the dressing to the chest wall, so be prepared to use a lot of tape. The third way of preventing reflux of air is to use an oblique chest tube tract when placing the tube. The obliqueness of the tract allows it to close in on itself when the tube is removed. Of course, if the tube is not fluctuating at removal, it is not necessary to be so careful about it.

PERICARDIAL CAVITY

The primary method of pericardial drainage is pericardiocentesis. Pericardiocentesis is almost always a diagnostic procedure. Sometimes, as in chronic effusion, it is therapeutic. In pericardial tamponade it must be followed by a thoracotomy for definitive treatment.

The technique of pericardiocentesis is illustrated in Fig. 10-11. The procedure can be done with the patient supine or sitting, depending on why it is being done and the patient's condition. Pericardiocentesis for the drainage of a pericardial effusion is best done with the patient in a sitting position. For most diagnostic purposes the supine position will do just as well. Use electrocardiographic monitoring of the patient. Prepare the upper abdomen and lower chest. Place drapes. Insert an 18- or 20-gauge needle through the skin just below and to the left of the xiphoid process. Use a short-bevel needle to avoid lacerating the heart. A small stab wound with a No. 11 blade helps avoid friction between the needle and the skin. Direct the needle up and to the patient's left, aiming for the posterior aspect of the left shoulder. The object of pericardiocentesis is to aspirate fluid without touching the heart. This is easier to do if the pericardium is distended with a chronic effusion. It can be difficult for acute bleeding or when the pericardium is not enlarged and the heart is immediately next to the pericardium. As in thoracentesis the danger point is when the last portion of fluid is being withdrawn. It is easy to lacerate the heart in an effort to get the last few milliliters of

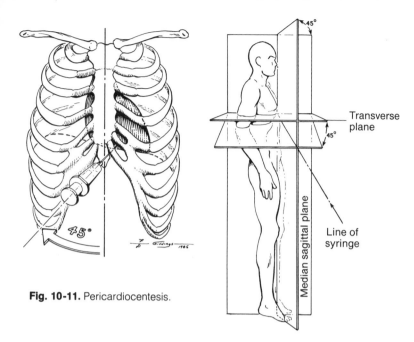

Fig. 10-11. Pericardiocentesis.

fluid. Even the most thorough pericardiocentesis, involving the use of a plastic catheter and multiple positions, will remove only about half of the pericardial fluid or blood that is present. For this reason pericardiocentesis demonstrating and relieving acute or chronic tamponade should be followed by an operation to relieve the problem permanently.

Pericardiocentesis is not used nearly as often as thoracentesis because it is more dangerous and the indications are less common. It should be approached with great caution and respect. Only rarely should the pericardial fluid be drained extensively; pericardial window or pericardiectomy is better for this purpose.

PERITONEAL CAVITY

Paracentesis, the needle aspiration of fluid from the peritoneal cavity, is a common procedure. In a large number of diseases fluid accumulates in the peritoneal cavity. There is one important difference between the pleural and peritoneal cavities: it is rarely necessary to leave any kind of indwelling tube in the peritoneal cavity and, in fact, it is undesirable. It is almost impossible to completely drain the peritoneal cavity. Furthermore, the surface area of the peritoneum is so large that any successful attempt would create a disasterous fluid loss. In fact, rapid aspiration of 1 to 2 L of peritoneal fluid is often followed by a large internal fluid loss as the peritoneal cavity refills. This is not to say that a paracentesis cannot be used for therapeutic purposes, but it has its dangers and should probably be used only with treatment for the underlying disorder. This contrasts sharply with the chest in which often the only necessary treatment for pleural effusion is thoracentesis.

The position of the patient during paracentesis depends on what is being done. If so much fluid is present that it interferes with breathing, the patient is usually more comfortable in a sitting position (Fig. 10-12). If the procedure is for diagnostic purposes only, the patient may be more comfortable lying down. Prepare a wide area of skin. Infiltrate a small skin wheal in the lower midline between the umbilicus and the pubis. Choosing this site is based on a number of considerations. The lower abdomen is usually the best site for paracentesis because it generally distends more with fluid. The lower midline is relatively thin. There are no large blood vessels that may be punctured, and there are normally no adhesions within the abdomen. Also the amount of preperitoneal fat in this particular area is small.

There are a number of reasons why the practitioner might wish to puncture the abdomen elsewhere. The most obvious reason is a previous surgical incision. If the patient has undergone a previous surgical procedure, there will be adhesions at the site of the incision. Also the bowel may be adherent to the abdominal wall. For that reason any previous incision site should be avoided. If the patient has had extensive pelvic surgery, it may be well to use the upper abdomen.

It is important to avoid puncturing the bowel, although this is probably a somewhat overrated hazard. If a 20- or 22-gauge needle is used, a puncture of the bowel will seal and heal spontaneously. It is not considered dangerous to puncture the mesentery, although it can cause bleeding or hematoma.

Once the site for paracentesis has been selected, the skin prepared, draped, and infiltrated with local anesthetic, insert a 20- or 22-gauge needle of appropriate length at right angles to the skin. A short-bevel needle should be used to minimize the

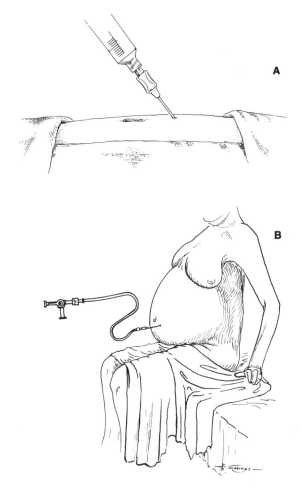

Fig. 10-12. Paracentesis. **A,** Placement of the needle in the lower midline. An over-needle cannula technique is best. **B,** Ideal position of patient, with drainage technique.

chance of lacerating the bowel. Use of short-bevel needles is made easier by nicking the skin with a knife prior to inserting the needle. An over-needle catheter or a through-needle catheter is especially desirable if a large amount of fluid is to be removed. The definitive method of draining the peritoneal cavity is with a dialysis catheter, as described in the next section under peritoneal lavage (Fig. 10-13).

Once the needle is in the peritoneal cavity and fluid can be aspirated, connect a three-way stopcock to the needle. Aspirate fluid without allowing air to enter the peritoneal cavity. This is not nearly as important a consideration as it is in the chest, but if fluid is to be removed, it would do little good to replace it with air. Remove no more than 1 L of fluid at a time. Refilling, as described earlier, may cause a patient to become hypotensive and show other signs of fluid volume deficit 1 to 2 hours after removing the fluid or even during removal of the fluid. It is better to aspirate fluid daily for 2 to 3 days rather than try to remove it all at one time.

Making a large needle hole should be avoided; therefore if a large needle is being used, run it obliquely through the abdominal wall. This is especially important in patients with ascites secondary to liver disease because the paracentesis site may ooze fluid for several days. A continued leak can lead to peritonitis.

Culdocentesis should be mentioned. In culdocentesis a needle is placed into the cul-de-sac immediately posterior to the cervix. The cul-de-sac is the most dependent portion of the peritoneal cavity. Bleeding that occurs anywhere in the peritoneal cavity will produce at least a small pool of blood in the cul-de-sac. Culdocentesis is especially useful in detecting ectopic pregnancies; however, it is a little difficult to perform and is probably best carried out by a gynecologist or general surgeon.

To do a culdocentesis, place a speculum in the vagina, visualize the cervix clearly, and then, using a cervical tenaculum or sponge forceps, lift the cervix out of the way. Place a long No. 18 needle into the cul-de-sac immediately posterior to the cervix. Care should be taken to avoid puncturing the rectum. If the test is positive, blood will be obtained immediately. The danger of culdocentesis is that if blood cannot be aspirated, persistent attempts may result in damage to adjacent structures. Culdocentesis is contraindicated after pelvic surgery because of the possibility that loops of bowel will be stuck down in the cul-de-sac.

The various techniques of needle aspiration from the abdominal cavity are simple enough to be performed by any physician. There is a danger of perforation of the bowel and bleeding from either the abdominal wall or the mesentery. However, with care these procedures are relatively safe and quite useful.

Peritoneal lavage

Peritoneal lavage is a technique for detecting intra-abdominal injury following blunt abdominal trauma. It allows the practitioner to diagnose intra-abdominal bleeding at an early stage, often before there is clinical evidence of blood loss.

Indications for peritoneal lavage are:

1. History of significant abdominal trauma
2. Evidence of abdominal trauma such as abrasions or contusions of the abdominal wall
3. Comatose patients with suspected abdominal trauma
4. Patients with neurologic deficits that obscure abdominal findings
5. Fractures of the lower ribs
6. Fractures of the pelvis
7. Patients with multiple trauma necessitating emergency surgery (to preclude circulatory collapse from missed intra-abdominal hemorrhage while under anesthesia)

Peritoneal lavage is indicated in penetrating wounds of the abdomen only if the wounds are not obviously in need of exploration.

Contraindications to peritoneal lavage are:

1. Urinary retention with a full bladder
2. Gravid uterus
3. Abdominal wall hematoma
4. Evidence of previous surgery in the lower abdomen

Lavage is ideally performed with a dialysis catheter placed through a small incision into the lower abdomen (Fig. 10-13). However, this type of catheter is not always available in the emergency department, so a through-needle catheter is often substituted.

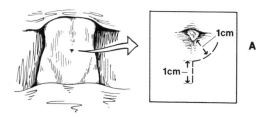

Fig. 10-13. Technique of peritoneal lavage. **A,** Position of skin incision. Inset shows detail of skin incision, which is intended to expose inferior umbilical ring and lower midline fascia. *Continued.*

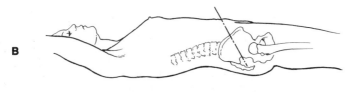

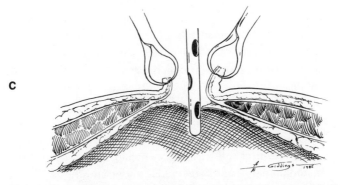

Fig. 10-13, cont'd. B, Insertion angle. The object is to direct the catheter into the pelvis. **C,** Placement. After exposing the fascia, make a short (3-4 mm) incision in lower midline fascia just at inferior umbilical ring. Grasping edges of incision with towel clamps, push dialysis catheter with trocar through peritoneum. Although a moderate amount of force is required to puncture the peritoneum, care must be taken that trocar does not penetrate more than two or three centimeters into abdomen. Then, remove trocar and advance catheter into pelvis along angle shown in **B.** Instill 1000 ml of lactated Ringer's solution into the abdomen, and allow it to drain out into the bottle.

After checking the abdomen for surgical scars and a gravid uterus, drain the bladder with a Foley catheter. Prepare and anesthetize the abdominal skin. Incise down to the inferior umbilical ring using a hockey-stick incision (Fig. 10-13). Dissect to the linea alba. Maintain perfect hemostasis to prevent contaminating the field with blood. Inject 1 ml of lidocaine agent with epinephrine through the fascia. Hold up the fascia with towel clips, incise, and insert the fascia down into the peritoneum. With firm control and upward traction on the peritoneum, make a small incision and insert the catheter into the peritoneal cavity using a rotary motion and directing it toward the sacrum. Thread the catheter into the hollow of the sacrum. Aspirate the contents through the catheter. If free blood, bile-stained contents, urine, or feces is returned, the diagnosis is made.

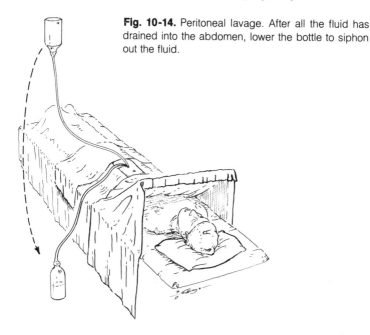

Fig. 10-14. Peritoneal lavage. After all the fluid has drained into the abdomen, lower the bottle to siphon out the fluid.

If the aspiration is negative, attach the catheter to an infusion system and administer 1 L of normal saline solution (15 ml/kg) in 20 minutes. While there is still fluid present in the tubing, place the infusion bottle on the floor and siphon out the abdominal fluid (Fig. 10-14). There should be at least 700 ml returned. Anything less would be an inadequate study. Test the returned fluid for culture and sensitivity, amylase, Gram stain, and cell count. After as much fluid as possible has been siphoned from the abdominal cavity, withdraw the catheter and close the skin with 4-0 nylon sutures.

The red cell count is the most important study. A cell count of more than 100,000 per ml is indication for surgical intervention. A red cell count between 50,000 per ml and 100,000 per ml is equivocal. A count below 50,000 is considered negative. In the case of a penetrating trauma the criteria are different. For stab wounds in the middle or lower abdomen a red cell count of over 100,000 per ml is indicative of intra-abdominal injury. But for wounds near the costal margin, between the nipples and the umbilicus, over 5,000 per ml is an indication for exploration. The reason for this is the greater chance of diaphragmatic injury. For

Fig. 10-15. Lumbar puncture.

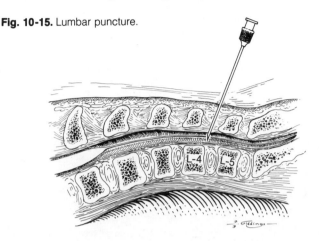

any gunshot wounds, a red cell count of over 5,000 per ml is an indication to operate.

The white blood cell count should also be done. If over 500 per ml, it is an indication for exploration. Amylase elevation, bacteria on Gram stain, or a (late) positive culture also mandate exploration.

If carefully performed, the peritoneal lavage is an extremely useful diagnostic technique that can both decrease the number of unnecessary abdominal explorations and enable the early diagnosis of intra-abdominal injuries.

LUMBAR PUNCTURE

Puncture of the subarachnoid space in the lumbar region is a widely used procedure (Fig. 10-15). Lumbar puncture is used to diagnose meningitis, detect subarachnoid hemorrhage, and induce spinal anesthesia. A related technique is used for epidural anesthesia, in which a needle is placed into the same general location, but not into the subarachnoid space, and local anesthetic agents are injected into the epidural space.

To perform lumbar puncture, position the patient either sitting up and leaning forward or on his side with his knees drawn up. These positions rotate the pelvis so that the sacrum is pulled anteriorly and the normal lumbar curvature is reversed. The spaces between the spinous processes are widened, and the subarachnoid space is most accessible. Prepare the skin over the lower lumbar spine and apply drapes. Draping is usually difficult because of the position of the patient. Identify the spinous process of T12 by the presence of the twelfth rib and the upper margin of the sacrum. By using these two landmarks it should be possible to identify each of the lumbar vertebrae. The spinal cord ends at the level of L2. Opposite the L3-4 and L4-5 intervertebral spaces is the cauda equina. The interspace between L4 and L5 is most often used for lumbar puncture. If L4-5 cannot be used, L3-4 may be used. The L2-3 interspace should *never* be used. The variation in position of the end of the spinal cord makes it possible that it will be injured by a needle placed through this interspace.

Use a 3-inch spinal needle, with the size depending on the procedure to be done. A No. 20 or 22 needle is adequate for most purposes. No. 18 spinal needles are also available, but many anesthesiologists prefer to use a No. 25 needle. The larger the needle, the larger the hole it will make through the dural membrane. Typically, a hole in the dural membrane will continue to leak spinal fluid for 1 to 2 days after the puncture. If enough spinal fluid leaks out, a severe headache will result. This so-called spinal headache is resistant to pain medication and can cause the patient considerable discomfort. Therefore in this procedure a small-diameter needle should be used, and the patient should be kept flat in bed for 12-24 hours following the procedure.

Insert the needle between the two spinous processes and angled upward 20 to 30 degrees. Advance the needle into the interspace. The first try may hit bone. If this happens, pull out the needle, use a slightly different angle, and push in again. If the angle is correct, the needle will go deep until it meets resistance. This resistance means that the needle is pressing against the vertebral body on the far side of the spinal canal. Pull the needle back slightly, take out the obturator, and check to see if spinal fluid drips freely from the needle. If it does not, the needle is probably too far to one side or another. If the needle is much too far to one side, pain may radiate down one leg or the other. Retract the needle a little further. If this still does not work, pull the needle all the way out, replace the obturator, and try again.

The most common error is placing the needle too far to one

side. The usual position is for the patient to be lying on his side with his knees drawn up. In general, this is an adequate position to use and is more comfortable for the patient than the sitting position. However, because the patient is on his side, slight angulations in his position may not be detected and the needle may be placed to one side or the other.

Once the subarachnoid space is entered, as shown by clear spinal fluid dripping freely from the end of the needle, measure the pressure. Pressures taken after removal of several milliliters of spinal fluid will not be as valid as the initial pressure. Connect a pressure manometer to the needle hub and read the pressure. Then ask the patient to strain down and then take a deep breath. If communication in the subarachnoid space between the lumbar area and the brain is free, the lumbar spinal fluid pressure area will rise on Valsalva maneuver and fall on inspiration.

Despite the danger of spinal headache, it is perfectly safe to remove 5 or 6 ml of fluid for diagnostic tests and microscopic examination. Note the color of the fluid. It should be crystal clear. Even a slight yellowish tinge is significant as evidence of an old subarachnoid hemorrhage. Occasionally a small blood vessel is punctured as the needle goes in and the first few drops of fluid come out bloody. After pressure is obtained, the fluid should be allowed to drip until clear. If the fluid remains bloody, the patient has had a recent subarachnoid hemorrhage. If the fluid is cloudy, there may be bacterial meningitis. Fluid should always be taken for cultures and tested for glucose.

● ● ●

In summary, diagnostic aspiration and therapeutic drainage of the major body cavities are commonly used in the modern hospital. Although each procedure has its own particular contra-indications and dangers, the biggest danger is the introduction of infection by the procedure itself. Rigid aseptic technique should be observed. All of these procedures should be done with adequate skin preparation, drape towels, gloves, mask, and meticulous attention to the details of aseptic technique. Although the procedures are relatively safe and are widely done by practitioners of all levels, they are followed by disaster if infection is introduced. All of these procedures should be treated with respect and used only for good reasons.

11

Bladder catheterization

Catheterization of the urinary bladder is an important and useful technique with which all physicians should become familiar. Indications for catheterization are as follows:

1. Inability to void secondary to:
   a. obstruction
   b. decreased bladder tone as seen in the postoperative patient
   c. neurologic diseases
2. To aid in the diagnosis of urological diseases
3. To provide a measurement of urinary output as in therapy of shock or fluid management problems

Although it is not an innocuous procedure, because of the incidence of urinary tract infection, the only real contraindication to catheterization is the presence of *urethral disruption*. This should be suspected in all cases of pelvic trauma. If there is blood at the meatus or a "high riding" prostate on rectal examination, the tentative diagnosis may be made. A urethrogram is necessary before attempting to catheterize the patient, if a urethral tear is suspected. This is obtained by injecting a small amount of radiopaque dye into the urethral meatus and obtaining an x-ray film to look for extravasation.

Practitioners should become familiar with the various types of catheterization trays used in their facilities. However, most facilities now use prepackaged disposable sets. Some of these sets contain all the necessary items for successful catheterization, and others, by design, lack certain items.

MALE CATHETERIZATION

The male patient should be lying in bed with his legs slightly abducted. Cleanse the entire genital area with the solution provided or with a liquid soap solution and cotton balls. As a final step, lift the penis, retract the foreskin, and thoroughly cleanse the meatal area. Rinse with a mild disinfectant or sterile water. While holding the penis erect, insert a well-lubricated catheter, advancing it gently until urine returns.

FEMALE CATHETERIZATION

Catheterization of the female is facilitated by having the patient fully abduct her legs and flex her knees. After initial cleansing of the genital area, gently spread the labia and thoroughly cleanse and rinse the introitus. With the labia still spread, locate the urethral meatus and gently insert the catheter.

SINGLE OR INTERMITTENT CATHETERIZATION

A single catheterization is usually all that is necessary for diagnostic and bacteriologic purposes. A No. 14 Fr (French) straight catheter (Fig. 11-1) is usually used for this procedure. Some male patients are difficult to catheterize because of hypertrophy of the prostate gland. A coudé catheter (Fig. 11-2) is especially designed for use under these circumstances since it is somewhat firmer than the regular catheter and is slightly curved at the tip. The point of the catheter should be held anteriorly as it is inserted so that the catheter can ride up over the enlarged posterior prostate.

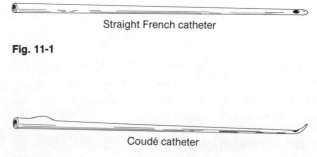

Straight French catheter

Fig. 11-1

Coudé catheter

Fig. 11-2

CONTINUOUS DRAINAGE

Use continuous urinary drainage if the urinary output is to be monitored or if the patient is (or will be) unable to void spontaneously. Use a No. 18 Fr Foley catheter in this situation (Fig. 11-3). This catheter is similar to the straight catheter, but it has an inflatable 10 ml balloon near the tip. Before inserting the catheter, make sure that the balloon will inflate and that there are no leaks. Insert the catheter in the same manner as a regular catheter, but insert it farther to ensure that the balloon does not lie in the urethra. Inflate the balloon by injecting 8 ml of saline solution into the balloon port. Newer Foley catheters have a self-sealing inflation port and are made of Silastic to decrease tissue reaction.

DIFFICULT CATHETERIZATION

Difficulty is frequently encountered while attempting catheterization, especially in the male. If the initial attempt at catheterization is unsuccessful, the following suggestions may be helpful:

1. Make sure the catheter is well lubricated and try again with the penis held rather firmly in the erect position
2. Inject 5 to 10 ml of sterile lubricant into the urethral meatus
3. Use a coudé catheter
4. If catheterization is urgent and a urologist is not immediately available, attempt the use of filiforms and followers or perform a percutaneous cystostomy

Fig. 11-3

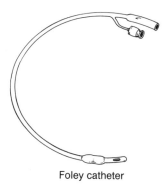

Foley catheter

Do *not* attempt further catheterization of the urethra. Remember that in trauma cases failure to catheterize the bladder might signify disruption of the urethra. A urethrogram should be obtained before proceeding further.

FILIFORMS AND FOLLOWERS

The filiform is a small woven guide that is relatively stiff. It should be used with extreme caution. Since the filiform is very small, it often passes quite easily. If it encounters an obstruction and does not pass into the bladder, leave the filiform in place and pass another one next to it. Repeat this process until one filiform finally enters the bladder. Then remove the other filiforms and attach the follower (Fig. 11-4). The filiform will act as a

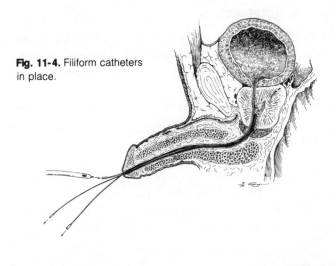

Fig. 11-4. Filiform catheters in place.

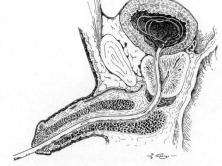

Fig. 11-5. Filiform catheter with follower in place.

guide and there should be no trouble advancing the follower into the bladder (Fig. 11-5). Tape the follower to the penis and connect it to a drainage system. Because the follower is rather stiff, it should not be left in place for a long period. A urologist or surgeon should be consulted to replace the follower with a standard catheter.

PERCUTANEOUS SUPRAPUBIC CYSTOSTOMY

When the urethra cannot be catheterized, percutaneous suprapubic cystostomy is very useful. It requires a relatively distended or palpable bladder. This technique should not be used in patients with known bladder abnormalities or marked hematuria. After adequate surgical preparation of the suprapubic area, insert a small trocar and cannula (or a large 14-gauge needle) from a point 2 cm above the pubis in the midline, and direct it toward the coccyx. When the bladder has been entered, withdraw the trocar and insert a small Silastic catheter through the cannula or needle (Fig. 11-6). After the catheter is inserted into the bladder, withdraw the cannula or needle, fix the catheter to the abdomen, and attach it to a drainage system.

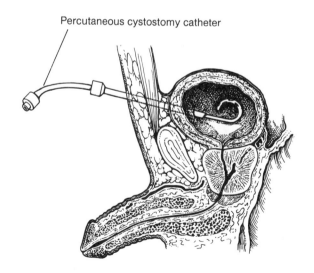

Percutaneous cystostomy catheter

Fig. 11-6. Bladder catheterization via percutaneous cystostomy.

• • •

Catheterization of the urinary bladder is not a completely benign procedure. Because it is associated with a high incidence of infection, meticulous aseptic techniques should be used during catheterization and the catheter should be removed as soon as possible.

12

Gastrointestinal intubation

All practitioners should know how to intubate the stomach or intestine. Though relatively simple, this procedure evokes a high level of patient anxiety and can be unpleasant for both patient and practitioner.

Intubation is indicated for:

1. Diagnosis—as in upper gastrointestinal bleeding
2. Lavage—as in suspected ingestion
3. Decompression—as in obstruction or prolonged ileus
4. Feeding

SHORT (NASOGASTRIC) TUBES

Short tubes are designed primarily to evacuate the stomach. This category includes three basic types.

The *Ewald tube* is a large tube for lavaging the stomach. It is also used to remove clots in gastric bleeding. It is often introduced through the mouth because of its size.

The *Levin tube* is the most common of the short tubes. This single-lumen tube is made of either rubber or plastic. Patients tolerate plastic tubes better than rubber tubes because they cause less pharyngeal and esophageal irritation. The average size is 14 Fr (5 mm in diameter). Single-lumen tubes require the administration of intermittent suction or gravity drainage because constant negative pressure sucks mucosa into the inlet holes, producing gastric mucosal damage.

The sump tube is a plastic double-lumen tube; the second, smaller lumen allows air to enter (Fig. 12-1). In theory, sump tubes can be used with constant suction, because the air coming down the smaller lumen should prevent obstruction or gastric mucosal damage. However, in practice, the sump tubes become blocked as often as single-lumen tubes, and produce as much gastric mucosal damage.

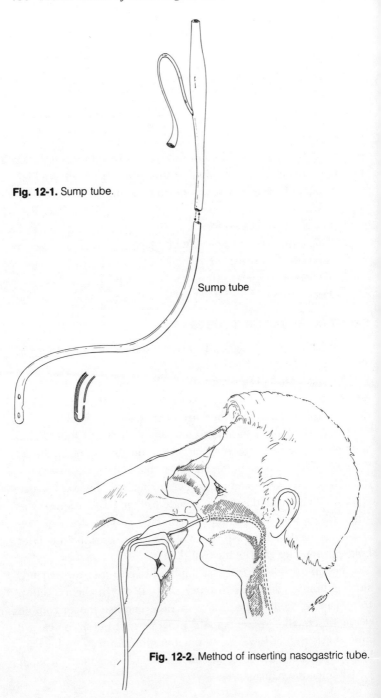

Fig. 12-1. Sump tube.

Sump tube

Fig. 12-2. Method of inserting nasogastric tube.

Insertion of nasogastric tubes

Most patients are extremely apprehensive about nasogastric intubation. Even in the hands of a skilled practitioner, it is at best unpleasant. A short explanation of the procedure will reassure the patient and decrease the problems associated with intubation.

The practitioner will begin by estimating the length of tube needed to reach the stomach. The distance from the bridge of the nose to the earlobe is added to the distance from the bridge of the nose to the tip of the xiphoid process. Most practitioners omit this step as they become familiar with the necessary length for intubation.

Provide the patient with cleansing tissues and an emesis basin. Lubricate 4 inches of the distal end of the tube with water-soluble jelly. Insert the tube slowly through the nostril and into the pharynx. At this point a gag reflex usually occurs. Withdraw the tube approximately 1 inch and encourage the patient to relax (Fig. 12-2).

Use only minimal pressure to pass the tube through the nares. If an obstruction is met, simply rotate the tube and it will usually pass the blockage without further resistance. Never force the tube. If the obstruction should persist, try to pass the tube through the other nostril.

Allow the patient to relax and tell him to swallow several times. At this time, give constant reassurance, and advance the tube steadily to its desired position. Have the patient swallow small sips of water through a straw, unless contraindicated.

Although some gagging is to be expected, even with successful passage, severe gagging and retching usually means that the tube is curling up in the esophagus. If this should occur, withdraw the tip of the tube back into the nasopharynx and allow the patient to relax again.

Coughing or wheezing attacks that occur during the attempt to pass the tube usually indicate that the trachea has been entered by mistake. Withdraw the tube into the nasopharynx before making another attempt at passage.

Nasogastric intubation is contraindicated in certain injuries. If the cribriform plate is fractured, a tube can be mistakenly passed from the nose into the skull. Therefore, in severe facial fractures, gastric tubes should be passed through the mouth.

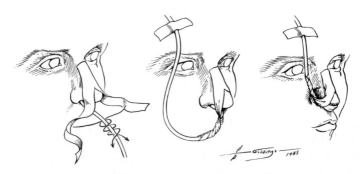

Fig. 12-3. Method used for securing nasogastric tube. Too tight a curve can cause pressure necrosis of the nares.

Once the tube has been passed, check it by aspiration to ensure proper placement in the stomach. Inject 5 to 10 ml of air while listening with a stethoscope placed on the epigastrium. A characteristic gurgle indicates stomach placement. Also, free return of gastric contents indicates successful intubation. Once proper placement is accomplished, secure the tube with tape (Fig. 12-3). Remember that a tube curled too sharply can put pressure on the nares and cause tissue necrosis. The tube may be pinned to the patient's gown to prevent excess tension during ambulation.

Care of nasogastric tubes

Nasogastric tubes should be irrigated with 30 ml of normal saline solution every 1 or 2 hours because they occlude frequently. A clogged tube can also be cleared by injecting it with 20 ml of air.

The intake and output of all patients undergoing nasogastric suction should be strictly controlled, because this is important for electrolyte replacement and is also an indication of possible or impending tube malfunction.

There is some discomfort associated with all nasogastric tubes. Good oral hygiene is essential to avoid inflammation of the parotid gland. Frequent rinsing of the mouth as well as good dental care are helpful. If allowed, the patient will usually appreciate sucking on ice chips. For severe irritation, having the patient gargle with saline or the use of viscous lidocaine is usually beneficial. Irritation of the opening of the eustachian tubes in

Fig. 12-4

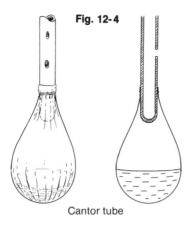

Cantor tube

the nasopharynx sometimes causes obstruction. A mild nasal decongestant can be helpful in preventing otitis.

Nasogastric tubes also irritate the gastric mucosa, especially along the lesser curvature, where small erosions and ulcerations are often present. Bleeding is commonly seen with prolonged intubation. As these tubes pass through the esophagogastric junction, they render the sphincter incompetent. Reflux of gastric contents into the esophagus commonly produces esophagitis.

Nasogastric tubes are undoubtedly helpful in the treatment of patients, however, their use is not without complication. Insertion of these tubes requires expertise, and constant attention is necessary for maintenance and proper function.

LONG TUBES

Long tubes are used primarily for intestinal decompression and infrequently for location of a bleeding site. With the aid of intestinal peristalsis, all long tubes can traverse the entire gastrointestinal tract. Therefore these tubes are of no value in patients without active peristalsis.

The *Cantor tube* (Fig. 12-4) is a single-lumen tube, much like a long Levin tube, with a latex balloon secured at the tip. This balloon is a reservoir for mercury and aids in the propulsion of the tube through the gastrointestinal tract. Prior to insertion in the nares, inject 5 to 8 ml of mercury into this balloon with a small-gauge needle. If the resulting mass is too large to pass through the nares, pass a tube with an empty balloon into the posterior pharynx, grasp it with a forceps, and deliver it through the mouth. Then inject the mercury into the balloon and have the patient swallow the balloon.

Intestinal intubation

Once a long tube has been inserted in the stomach, peristalsis and gravity are required for its passage through the pylorus and into the gastrointestinal tract. Proper positioning of the tip of the tube is a prerequisite for this to occur. The tube should be positioned, if possible, with fluoroscopy. A tube that is curled within the stomach, with its tip in the fundus, will not pass. Proper positioning of the patient will aid in passing the tube through the pylorus. The patient should be in a semi-Fowler's position, inclined toward the right side, or in a right decubitus position.

Once through the pylorus, the tube will be propelled through the small bowel by peristalsis. The tube should not be securely attached to the nose for this reason. An x-ray film provides the best confirmation of successful intestinal intubation.

Care of long tubes

Long tubes require the same type of care used for nasogastric tubes. In fact, because of the "wick effect" of the tube, oral hygiene should be even more vigorous. Allow long tubes to progress until the point of obstruction is reached. If the obstruction is relieved, the tube may traverse the entire gastrointestinal tract. As soon as the patient begins passing flatus and having bowel movements, stop the progress of the tube by securing it to the nose.

Removal of long tubes

A long tube should be removed slowly and in steps. Withdraw it 8 to 12 inches, while firmly securing the tube to the nose. In 2 hours, withdraw it another 12 inches. Repeat this process until the tip of the tube is in the stomach; then it can be completely withdrawn. This step-by-step removal avoids "telescoping" of the bowel on the tube.

If the tip of the tube has passed the ileocecal valve, it may be difficult to withdraw it. If difficulty is encountered, it is wise to cut the tube off at the nose and let it pass naturally through the rectum.

FEEDING TUBES

For the patient who cannot eat enough, but who has a functioning bowel and intestine, feeding via a gastric tube is indicated. There are a number of small Silastic tubes made for this purpose, with sizes ranging from 8 to 12 French. The tubes are mercury-weighted at the tip to allow them to be swallowed. Some tubes are designed to stay in the stomach; other tubes are longer and designed to pass into the intestines.

The technique of insertion is simple. Lubricate the tube lightly with water-soluble jelly. Then introduce it through the nose. The tube is too flimsy to pass, so the patient must swallow it. Verify the position by injecting air into the tube (see p. 182). If it is desirable for the tube to reach the intestines, put the patient on his right side to encourage passage into the duodenum. For final confirmation of position, an x-ray film is necessary.

13

Airway maintenance

Back in the good old days of the house call and the horse and buggy, things were really much simpler. If a patient could not breathe, he died. Simple. Sometimes physicians did tracheostomies, but even then the patient had to be able to breathe for himself. Anesthesia has made possible endotracheal intubation, the treatment of polio brought techniques of ventilation, and, finally, the past decade of experience with volume-cycled ventilators has enabled us to keep patients alive when their lungs are in acute failure. All of this has placed an ever-increasing emphasis on access to the patient's airway (Fig. 13-1).

PHARYNGEAL AIRWAY

When a patient is supine and unconscious, the tongue tends to fall back into the oropharynx (Fig. 13-2, A). This obstructs the airway. A pharyngeal airway, placed into the mouth and oropharynx to support the tongue, relieves the obstruction (Fig. 13-2, B). In the hospital it is commonly used in conjunction with an endotracheal tube. But in an emergency situation, it can be life-saving in itself.

OROTRACHEAL INTUBATION

This basic technique for airway access is the first step in most forms of ventilatory support, including general anesthesia. Endotracheal tubes for adults generally have a balloon cuff on the end to occlude the airway (Fig. 13-3, A). This is the so-called low-pressure cuff; when the cuff is inflated, it is much larger than the trachea. When partly inflated, to a relatively low pressure, it will still occlude the airway. Any balloon cuff tends to produce erosion of the tracheal mucosa; the low-pressure cuff minimizes the damage. For infants, the use of the balloon is generally not

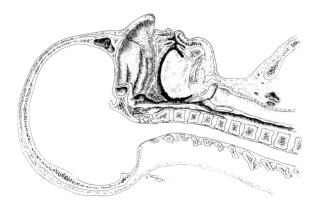

Fig. 13-1. Normal airway, sagittal section.

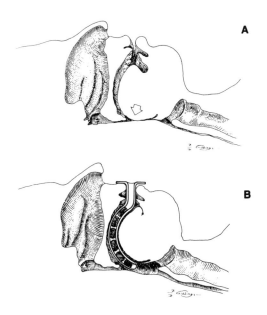

A

B

Fig. 13-2. A, In the unconscious patient, the tongue falls back into the oro-pharynx, blocking the airway. **B,** Pharyngeal airway in place.

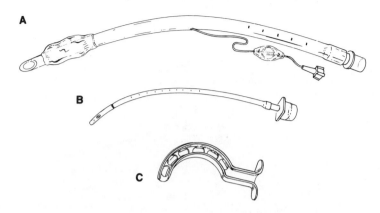

Fig. 13-3. Endotracheal tubes. **A,** Adult. **B,** Infant. **C,** Pharyngeal airway.

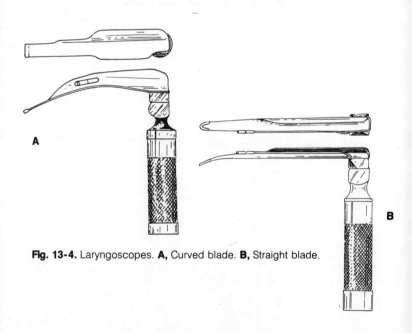

Fig. 13-4. Laryngoscopes. **A,** Curved blade. **B,** Straight blade.

necessary, because the hypopharyngeal soft tissues and the larynx will occlude the airway around the tube.

As noted in Chapter 2, there are two types of laryngoscopes available, the straight-blade and the curved-blade (Fig. 13-4). Both types are widely used. Anesthesiologists, who use them

Fig. 13-5. A, Curved blade technique. **B,** Placement of tube with curved blade laryngoscope.

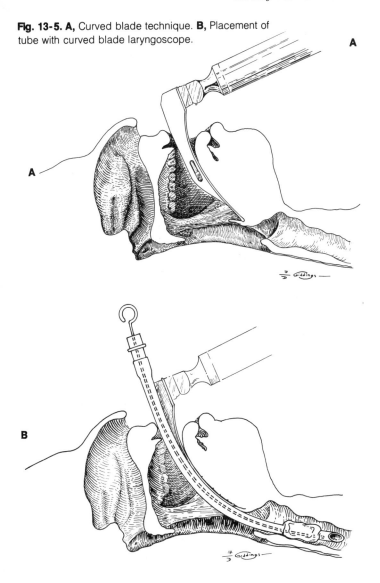

every day, generally prefer the curved-blade instrument. But many other practitioners find that the straight-blade type is somewhat easier to use.

To place an endotracheal tube with the curved-blade laryngoscope, insert the rounded tip into the hypopharynx in such a way that it lies at the base of the tongue, just anterior to the epiglottis (Fig. 13-5, *A*). Then lift straight up, pulling the tongue out of the

Fig. 13-6. Straight blade technique.

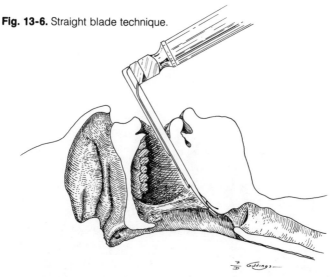

way. Looking down along the instrument, it should be possible to see the epiglottis and, by lifting the laryngoscope, the arytenoid cartilages. Pass the tube along the blade. Guide its tip anterior to the arytenoid cartilages and between the vocal cords into the trachea (Fig. 13-5, *B*). A metal obturator keeps the soft plastic tube curved, making it much easier to guide the tube through the vocal cords. Sometimes the cords will close tightly causing *laryngospasm.* If this happens, ease the tube gently up against the vocal cords and, using the tapered tip to wedge the cords apart, pass between them. Be gentle; too much force may cause dislocation of an arytenoid cartilage.

To insert an endotracheal tube with the straight-blade laryngoscope, lift the epiglottis up and out of the way with the tip (Fig. 13-6). It should then be possible to see the vocal cords. Pass the tube along the instrument and into the larynx. One of the difficulties with the straight-blade instrument is that although it gives a better view of the vocal cords, this view becomes completely obscured when the tube is passed into the larynx. However, this instrument is somewhat easier to learn to use than the curved-blade laryngoscope.

After passing the tube, grasp it firmly with one hand and remove the laryngoscope; then remove the obturator with the other hand, put in a pharyngeal airway to prevent the patient's

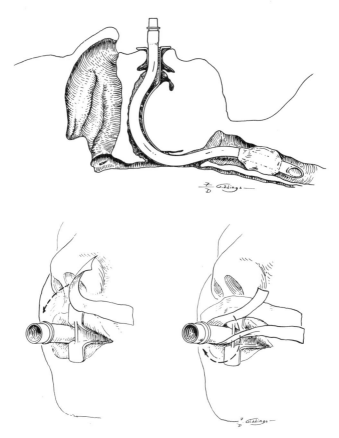

Fig. 13-7. Endotracheal tube in place, with pharyngeal airway, showing details of securing the tube and airway with adhesive tape.

biting down on the tube, and tape the tube in place (Fig. 13-7). Cut the plastic tube 1 to 2 inches from the patient's lips and place the adapter in the shortened tube. Connect the tube to the anesthesia bag, or ventilator, and inflate the balloon to the minimum necessary to occlude the airway. For future use, note the volume of air required. The balloon pressure, if measured, should be less than 40 mm Hg. Finally, listen over both sides of the chest to ensure that the tube has not been placed into the right main bronchus. In any emergency intubation, a chest x-ray film should be obtained as soon as possible to ensure proper positioning.

An endotracheal tube can be left in place for days or even weeks. However, with prolonged intubation, three difficulties occur. First, the vocal cords may become damaged. Second, the balloon may damage the trachea, leading to late stricture formation, tracheomalacia, tracheal to innominate artery fistula, or tracheoesophageal fistula. Third, the tube may become occluded by inspissated secretions, especially in infants. The last problem can be prevented by changing the tube periodically. Nonetheless, the long and relatively narrow endotracheal tube often makes it difficult to aspirate secretions.

NASOTRACHEAL INTUBATION

The technique for nasotracheal intubation is very different from orotracheal intubation, and it is used only in patients with spontaneous respiratory effort. A No. 7 tube should be used. Lubricate both the tube and the nose with lidocaine jelly. Before passing the tube, mark off a distance the same as that from the anterior nares to the earlobe. Pass the tube into the nares, down along the floor of the nose, and into the nasopharynx and pharynx. When the tube is advanced to the mark, its tip will lie in the lower pharynx. Then advance the tube slowly, with gentle pressure on the larynx. The patient's breathing will be heard through the tube. Try to obtain maximum breath sounds by advancing the tube and manipulating the larynx with the other hand. The tip of the tube should be just in the larynx at this point. Continue to advance the tube gently into the larynx, and through the cords (Fig. 13-8). If the tube fails to pass, withdraw it into the pharynx and try again. If all else fails, and if the patient is not awake, use a

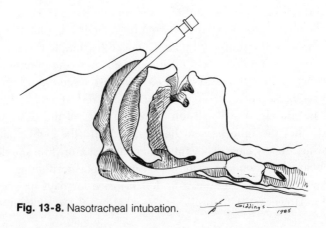

Fig. 13-8. Nasotracheal intubation.

laryngoscope to visualize the larynx. Pass the tube into the larynx with *Robinson forceps.*

The major advantage of the nasotracheal tube is that it is better tolerated by the awake patient. The major problem is that the tube is longer and smaller to suction through, and blocks more easily. However, for the awake or semi-awake patient, it is often the best means of airway access.

TRACHEOSTOMY

Tracheostomy, in one form or another, has been around for several thousand years. Galen warned against it in Roman days. So great was his influence that it was little used during the Middle Ages and not widely used until the last century. It is an excellent procedure when done properly and for specific indications.

There are three indications for tracheostomy. First, a tracheostomy is more convenient and more comfortable than an endotracheal tube for a patient who will be receiving ventilator therapy for more than 1 or 2 weeks, or who will be comatose for a long time. Second, suctioning and coughing are more effective through a short, large tracheostomy tube, especially for the patient who has large amounts of tracheobronchial secretions. Third, tracheostomy is indicated if the larynx is obstructed.

Tracheostomy is not a very good emergency procedure. If a patient stops breathing, brain damage occurs in 4 minutes. It is difficult to obtain instruments and perform a tracheostomy within this time frame. The first priority should be to use a pharyngeal airway, mask, and bag to help the patient breathe. The second priority should be to put in an endotracheal tube. Once the tube is in place, there is time to do a tracheostomy. Only if it is impossible to ventilate the patient with a bag and mask should a tracheostomy be done as an emergency. Note that only the last indication may be considered a true emergency. Even with laryngeal obstruction, it should be possible to use a needle cricothyroidotomy with jet ventilation rather than a tracheostomy (see next section).

The first two indications are relative. In burns, for example, a tracheostomy should not be considered. Even if the skin over the neck is unburned, the skin will become contaminated from the

burn wound and the tracheostomy site will usually become infected. Immunosuppressed patients tolerate tracheostomy
poorly. In such situations prolonged use of endotracheal tubes
may be preferred to tracheostomy.

Two techniques for tracheostomy are in common use: cricothyroidotomy and low tracheostomy. Cricothyroidotomy is probably dangerous for long-term use and should be used only as an
emergency procedure. Neither type of tracheostomy is a procedure for the inexperienced. While it is simple for the trained
surgeon, the low tracheostomy, especially, can be terrifying to
the uninitiated. When doing either type of tracheostomy for the
first time, it seems that everything that is cut bleeds. Cricothyroidotomy is relatively fast and simple, but it has to be done
without hesitation, and with sure knowledge of where the structures are.

Cricothyroidotomy is the easier of the two procedures (Fig.
13-9). After the skin has been prepared and the field draped,
grasp the larynx with one hand. With the other hand, palpate the
thyroid cartilage and cricoid cartilage immediately below it.
Using a scalpel with a No. 15 blade, stab into the skin transversely in the midline. Cut through the cricothyroid membrane

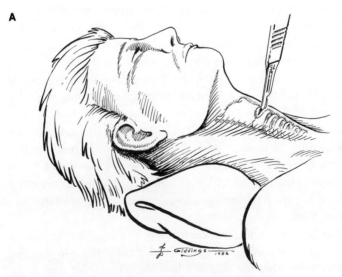

Fig. 13-9. Cricothyroidotomy. **A,** Incision.

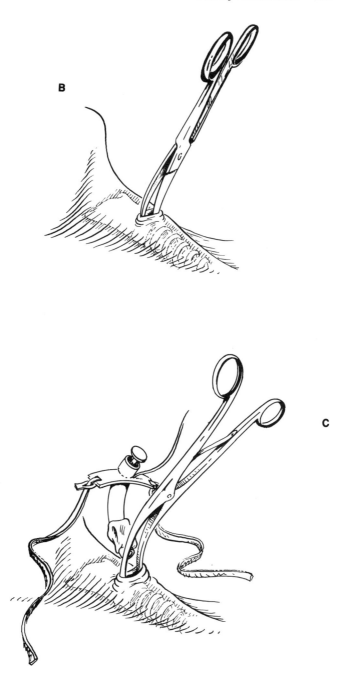

Fig. 13-9, cont'd. B, Spreading the opening. **C,** Placing the tube.

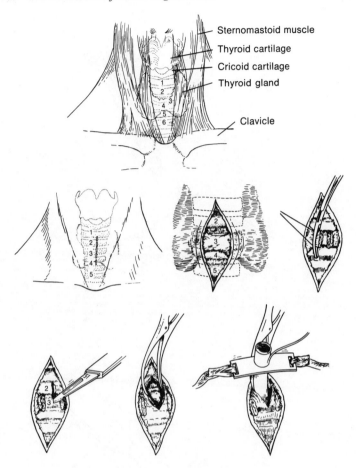

Fig. 13-10. Tracheostomy.

and into the larynx. The incision should be only 6 or 7 mm long. Pass a pair of blunt-pointed scissors into the wound and spread transversely. Using a large Kelly clamp or a Trousseau-Jackson dilator, spread along the long axis of the trachea. Force the cricoid and thyroid cartilages apart to permit an 8 mm tube to be placed through the space. (Obviously a smaller tube is needed for children.) Since the cricothyroid membrane measures, on the average, 9 mm by 3 cm, this should be possible. An experienced surgeon can do a cricothyroidotomy in 30 seconds.

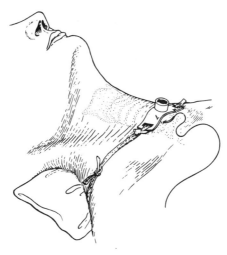

Fig. 13-11. Securing the tracheostomy tube.

The standard tracheostomy is performed in a similarly prepared and draped field. An endotracheal tube should be in place. Position a folded sheet under the shoulders. Make a short vertical incision in the midline just above the suprasternal notch (Fig. 13-10). A horizontal incision is thought to produce better cosmetic results; however, either one leaves a fairly ugly scar. Carry the incision down through the midline fascia between the strap muscles. When dissecting, use forceps to lift the tissues before cutting them. Never cut down into the neck. Retractors are usually not necessary. Palpate the trachea and identify both the cricoid cartilage and the first ring. The tracheostomy should be placed at the level of the second and third rings. Usually, the thyroid isthmus overlies these. Identify the isthmus, divide it between clamps, and ligate it with sutures; or displace the isthmus superiorly. Then incise the second and third rings in the midline. This usually punctures the balloon of the endotracheal tube. Dilate the tracheal wound with a clamp or a Trousseau-Jackson dilator and insert the tracheostomy tube. Use the largest tube that will fit; airway resistance will be least, suctioning easiest, and minimal balloon inflation necessary.

Secure the tube in two ways (Fig. 13-11). First, sew the

plastic flaps of the tracheostomy tube to the skin on either side of the incision with 2-0 or larger suture. Second, tie the tapes attached to the tube around the neck after the roll under the shoulders has been removed. Place a dressing around the tracheostomy tube to protect the wound. The wound should not be sutured.

Nearly all tracheostomy tubes available are disposable plastic with low-pressure cuffs (Fig. 13-12). For infants, small, uncuffed Silastic tubes are used. Silastic is minimally reactive and bends with movement. However, the wall thickness of Silastic tubes is greater than that of plastic tubes.

Complications of tracheostomy are of three kinds: operative, indwelling, and late or postextubation. Operative complications are injuries to adjacent structures: the carotid artery or jugular vein may be incised; the recurrent laryngeal nerve may be cut; the thyroid may bleed; the back wall of the trachea may be injured. A pneumothorax may be caused by injury to the apices of the pleura (from aspiration of air into the mediastinum through the open wound, or rupture through the thin mediastinal pleura into the pleural cavity). Most of these problems can be avoided

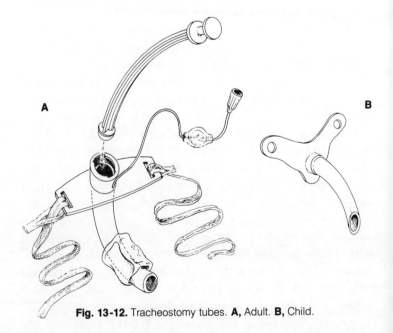

A

B

Fig. 13-12. Tracheostomy tubes. **A,** Adult. **B,** Child.

by doing the procedure with an endotracheal tube in place and with adequate lighting, assistance, instruments, anesthesia, and time.

Most complications of tracheostomy are usually related to the balloon. However, the tip of the tube can also cause direct injury. The tube may become pushed down the right bronchus, or plugged with secretions. These problems are considerably worse in infants. In premature infants, tube obstruction is a significant cause of death, and dislodgment, especially early, can also be fatal. Rupture of the balloon in a patient receiving ventilatory therapy can be a major crisis. Finally, the tracheostomy site may become infected, which can lead to mediastinitis.

Late complications are tracheal stenosis and tracheomalacia. These can occur with either endotracheal tubes or tracheostomy. Balloon damage to the trachea begins with mucosal erosion and necrosis and progresses to pressure necrosis and destruction of the cartilages. When this happens, the site of the balloon may heal with granulation tissue, ultimately producing a fibrous stenosis, and with loss of cartilage in the tracheal wall, producing tracheomalacia. Stenosis produces obstruction on both inspiration and expiration; tracheomalacia produces difficulty on inspiration only. A similar process, with the same results, may occur at the tracheostomy site. This is especially true if the tracheostomy becomes infected. Treatment requires resection of the damaged segment and reanastomosis of the normal portions of the trachea. Although symptomatic narrowing is uncommon, a high percentage of patients who have had long-term endotracheal intubation or tracheostomies are left with subclinical stenosis.

NEEDLE AND JET INSUFFLATION

For temporary use, such as in trauma, a large No. 14 or 16 needle may be used to puncture the cricothyroid membrane. This can be connected to a jet ventilator. The ventilator is nothing more than a tank containing high pressure oxygen or air, and a thumb-operated intermittent valve. The larynx must remain open proximally to allow exhalation. Good ventilation *in the normal lung* can be obtained. This needle and jet insufflation method is best for problems such as head injury and upper airway obstruction. It may not provide adequate ventilation for patients with chest injuries, especially when the chest is crushed. It is an extremely valuable technique in emergencies.

SUCTION AND TRACHEAL LAVAGE

Since the patient usually cannot expectorate his own secretions, especially if an endotracheal tube is in place, it is necessary to do it for him (Fig. 13-13). Basic technique involves one hand gloved, one hand nonsterile. Pick up the suction catheter, already connected to the suction line, using the gloved hand. Disconnect the ventilator with the ungloved hand and put in the catheter. Occlude the side hole in the suction catheter with the ungloved hand. Collect specimens in a suction trap. Instill 5 to 10 ml of sterile saline into the catheter to wash the trachea and bronchi. Repeat three or four times, aspirating after each instillation.

Avoid aspirating for too long, because the patient is not breathing well. If all of the inspired air is removed, the patient will become hypoxic. The best technique for determining the correct length of time is for the practitioner to hold his breath while aspirating.

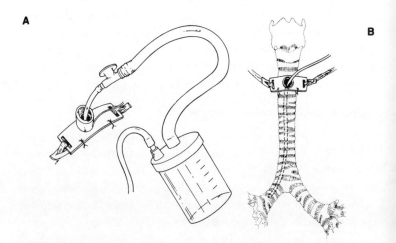

Fig. 13-13. A, Suction trap for sputum collection. **B,** Suction catheter placed in right bronchus.

The catheter normally passes into the right main bronchus (Fig. 13-12, *B*). The left bronchus, which comes off at a sharper angle, is harder to enter. Turning the patient's head does not help. If suctioning is being done through a tracheostomy, the tracheostomy tube can be directed to the left and the catheter will usually pass down the left bronchus. When suctioning through an endotracheal tube, the best technique is to remove the catheter, notice its natural curve, and wind the tip tightly around a finger in the same direction to increase the curve in the tip of the catheter. This curve will be transient, but most plastic catheters will "form" sufficiently well for this purpose. Rubber catheters are available with an angled tip.

Nasotracheal suction is a basic technique of medical care. It is used in a patient who is retaining secretions (Fig. 13-14). Pass the tube through the nose, just as in nasotracheal intubation. As the tube passes into the hypopharynx, tilt the patient's head back. Place the plastic tube so that its natural curve will direct the tip away from the esophagus and into the trachea. With proper positioning, the tube will pass. If it does not, vary the head position. In difficult cases, use a tube with an angled tip. Passage is signalled by air whistling in and out of the tube with breathing. Connect the suction tube and do tracheal suction as described above. Lavage through the tube is useful. It is difficult to reach the left bronchus with this technique; not impossible, just difficult.

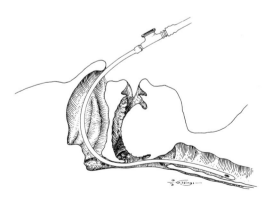

Fig. 13-14. Nasotracheal suction, cross section.

OXYGEN AND HUMIDITY

For a patient breathing on his own, but with respiratory problems, care should be taken to both humidify and enrich the enspired air. Humdification is best done with an ultrasonic vaporizer; the common wall-mounted humidifier is not adequate, unless it has a heater to increase the humidity. Humidification is essential for the patient with an endotracheal or tracheostomy tube who has lost the normal humidification of the upper airway, and it is often desirable for the nonintubated patient. Oxygen is also beneficial, although the inspired concentration should be kept below 40% to minimize oxygen toxicity to the lungs. The exact reason why oxygen is beneficial is not always clear, but it does help and should, in most instances, be given to patients with respiratory difficulty.

• • •

Airway maintenance techniques are basic to the care of the acutely ill patient. In an average intensive care unit, half the patients will require respiratory support and the rest will require periodic nasotracheal suction. Whatever their disease process, the patients will often recover if their airway and respiratory care is good, and they will die if it is not.

14

Cardiopulmonary resuscitation

One of the oddities of our day is that the local fireman may have a better knowledge of *cardiopulmonary resuscitation* (CPR) than the average health professional. Specialists such as the anesthesiologist, the thoracic surgeon, and the intensive care unit nurse deal with CPR on an everyday basis. However, for most of us, CPR must be learned and relearned constantly, so we will know the techniques when we need them.

There are two kinds of CPR. Basic cardiac life support is taught to paramedics, emergency medical technicians, and firemen. It consists of artificial ventilation and external cardiac massage and can be applied in any emergency situation. Advanced cardiac life support is taught to physicians and nurses, and is available only in medical facilities. It includes electrical defibrillation, intravenous fluids, drugs, and ventilators.

To a great extent, *Basic Cardiac Life Support* (BCLS) and *Advanced Cardiac Life Support* (ACLS) are defined in terms of their training courses. These courses are given through the American Heart Association, which certifies both providers and instructors. For detailed instruction in BCLS and ACLS, these courses should be taken. A brief outline of the basic principles follows.

CARDIAC ARREST

Cardiac arrest has occurred when a patient stops breathing and has no femoral or carotid pulse. If someone suffers a cardiac arrest in your presence, you can make two assumptions. First, the patient has enough oxygen to continue brain function for 4 minutes. Second, the heart is in one of three rhythms: standstill, ventricular fibrillation, or ventricular tachycardia. A precordial thump may be successful in starting the heart working again. This is accomplished by a firm blow to the lower half of the

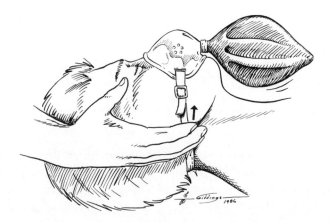

Fig. 14-1. Jaw thrust. Push the angle of the mandible forward with the fingers to clear the airway. A pharyngeal airway is helpful. Use a breathing mask, as shown, if available, or use mouth-to-mouth ventilation.

sternum, delivered with the closed fist, from a distance of 12 to 18 inches above the chest. This mechanically stimulates the heart and may convert ventricular tachycardia or standstill to normal rhythm.

Airway control

The first step in BCLS or ACLS is *airway control.* First, clear the airway. Swab vomitus and secretions from the pharynx. Lift the chin and mandible forward to move the tongue out of the airway (Fig. 14-1). Insert a pharyngeal airway, if one is available. Cardiac arrest can be produced by airway blockage alone. The "restaurant arrest" is classically caused by a piece of meat in the larynx. The immediate treatment is the *Heimlich maneuver.* Grab the patient around the lower chest in a bear hug and give a quick, forceful squeeze. This forces 200 to 400 ml of air from the chest and will dislodge a laryngeal obstruction.

Ventilation

The second step is *breathing.* Occlude the nose and apply mouth-to-mouth ventilation (Fig. 14-2). If mask, bag, and oxygen are available, use them (Fig. 14-1); however, ventilation of the patient should begin at once, without waiting for mechanical aids.

Fig. 14-2. Mouth-to-mouth ventilation.

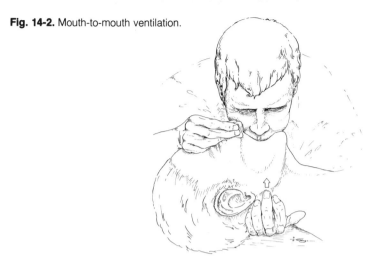

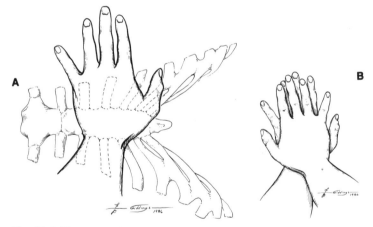

Fig. 14-3. Placement of hands for external cardiac massage.

External cardiac massage

The third step is *external cardiac massage*. With the patient supine, preferably on a flat, hard surface, kneel by the patient, place the heel of the hand on the lower third of the sternum, and sharply depress it 3 to 5 cm. Use both hands, one over the other (Fig. 14-3). This compresses both ventricles between the ster-

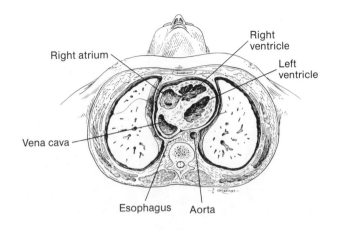

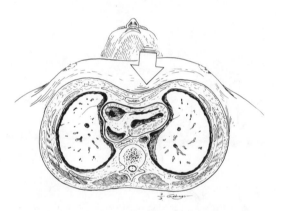

Fig. 14-4. Mechanics of external cardiac massage.

num and the spine, driving blood out into the pulmonary artery and aorta (Fig. 14-4). After pushing the sternum down, hold it down for a moment and then release, so that the compression phase is about as long as the release phase. The rate of massage should be 60 per minute. For infants, place one hand behind the child and use two fingers of the other hand to depress the sternum, at a rate of 100 per minute (Fig. 14-5).

Even under ideal circumstances, cardiac output during external massage is no more than half the normal rate. Blood pressure is 100/0, with a mean of 40 to 50 mm Hg. Cerebral blood flow is 30% to 40% of normal. It is common practice to "monitor" the external massage by palpating the femoral pulse. This is

Fig. 14-5. External cardiac massage in infants.

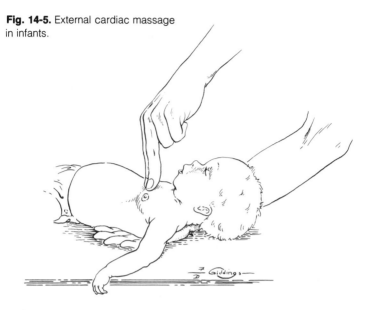

somewhat misleading. The pulse is basically a pressure wave traveling down the aorta and may be present even with a very low cardiac output.

Internal cardiac massage

Under adverse conditions—severe crushed chest, cardiac tamponade, cardiac wounds, pectus carinatum, or severe emphysema—external massage is ineffective. If external massage is ineffective, internal massage is indicated. For the trained surgeon this is quite easy. Incise below the left breast from the sternum to the anterior axillary line. Enter the chest through the interspace. Cut the upper costal cartilage next to the sternum. Incise the pericardium with scissors, avoiding the phrenic nerve. Put one hand under the heart and compress it against the sternum or put the other hand anterior to the heart and compress the heart between the two hands.

Internal massage is quite effective. Ventricular fibrillation can often be reverted by internal massage alone. But it takes an expert to do a thoracotomy in 1 to 2 minutes, and the chest must later be closed in the operating room. This technique can be life-saving; however, it is not for untrained personnel.

Coordination between ventilation and massage is not necessary. Ventilate once every six cardiac cycles. External massage should be applied continuously without stopping for ventilation.

One person can carry out both ventilation and external massage, although it is nearly impossible to keep it up for more than a few minutes. Two people can continue indefinitely, by trading places. Hopefully, the patient will respond to basic support. Ventricular tachycardia and ventricular standstill may revert to normal rhythm, although ventricular fibrillation usually will not. Therefore the next step is to use advanced support as quickly as possible.

ADVANCED LIFE SUPPORT

First, recruit more people. A team of four to six is required. In addition to the two people performing ventilation and external massage, one is needed for the ECG-defibrillator, one to start the intravenous fluids, and one to manage the drugs. The most experienced physician present, whatever his role in the arrest, should be in charge; half a dozen people running in all directions will rarely produce a successful outcome.

Determine the cardiac status with an ECG or cardiac monitor. Newer ECG-defibrillator units have cardiac monitors built in and will record the ECG from the defibrillator paddles. If ventricular fibrillation or ventricular tachycardia is present, defibrillate immediately. Apply the external defibrillator paddles, well-coated with conductive cream, to the skin over the base and apex of the heart (Fig. 14-6). Defibrillate the heart using 200 to 300 joules of electricity. If two shocks in quick succession fail to work, the heart is probably hypoxic; reapply massage and ventilation for 2 to 3 minutes and try again.

Meanwhile, intravenous access should be obtained. A peripheral line is easiest to start. Saphenous cutdown is useful if all veins are collapsed. A central catheter allows rapid access to the heart for giving drugs, but inserting it is difficult while external massage is being performed. Insert a central line as soon as the massage can be stopped.

The first drug should be one ampule (50 mEq) of sodium bicarbonate administered intravenously. If blood gas measurements are available, they should be used to guide subsequent bicarbonate administration; otherwise, give 25 mEq every 10 to

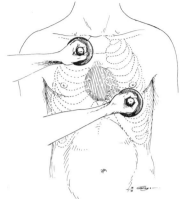

Fig. 14-6. Placement of external defibrillator paddles.

15 minutes. All patients become acidotic, but the degree varies greatly and rules of thumb are not reliable.

The next drug used depends on the cardiac rhythm. For fibrillation or tachycardia, give 1 mg/kg of lidocaine, followed by an infusion of 2 to 4 mg/min. Other ventricular antiarrhythmic drugs are procainamide and bretylium tosylate. Verapamil is useful for supraventricular arrhythmias.

If cardiac standstill is present, use epinephrine (0.5 mg bolus, or 5 ml of 1:10,000 dilution). This drug is also useful if defibrillation produces normal sinus rhythm but low cardiac output. Calcium chloride, 1 gm (10 ml of 10% solution), may improve myocardial contractility. Isoproterenol (1 to 5 μg/min) or dopamine (0.5 to 4 mg/min) may be useful.

Epinephrine is sometimes given as a direct intracardiac injection. The technique is very similar to pericardiocentesis (Fig. 14-7). The subxiphoid is probably the best approach, because it avoids the lung and the anterior descending coronary artery. Puncture the skin to the left of the xiphoid, using a 20-gauge, 3-inch needle. Aim toward the back of the patient's left shoulder and advance the needle. Aspirate continuously. Immediately on drawing blood, inject the drug and quickly remove the needle.

There are two other, less desirable, routes of direct cardiac puncture, the *apical* and the *anterior* approaches. The apex may be punctured by inserting the needle below the left breast in the midclavicular line, going over the rib, and then aiming toward the right shoulder. Although this approach avoids the coronary

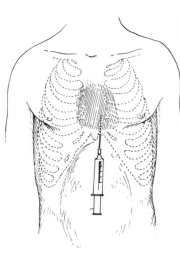

Fig. 14-7. Technique of cardiac puncture for intracardiac injection.

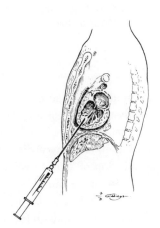

arteries, it may puncture the lung and is less accurate. In the
anterior approach, direct the needle over the fifth rib anteriorly
to the left of the sternum and push straight back. This method is
dangerous and should not be used. For example, with this approach, one may hit the internal mammary artery, lung, or anterior descending coronary artery.

In fact, all of these approaches are dangerous. Because they
are essentially stab wounds of the heart, they can all produce
bleeding and cardiac tamponade. Only if the heart is in standstill
and an intravenous route is not available should this route be
used, and then only once.

Systemic pressor agents

Systemic pressor agents can be used to increase the blood
pressure on the theory that the cerebral and cardiac vessels will
be preferentially perfused. Norepinephrine is often used; however, the mixed stimulators, epinephrine and dopamine, are

probably better. Peripheral constrictor agents are hazardous because they decrease flow.

Judicious use of fluids may be helpful. The patient suffering from a cardiac arrest is essentially in cardiogenic shock, so fluids should be given cautiously. However, the administration of 500 to 1000 ml of saline or Ringer's lactate may increase circulating volume and cardiac output.

An endotracheal tube should be inserted. A mechanical ventilator may be used; however, a bag usually produces better ventilation during external cardiac massage.

If cardiac standstill persists, temporary transcutaneous or transvenous pacing wires may be successful in producing a cardiac rhythm. These wires may be left in place for several days.

If all else fails, open thoracotomy, as described previously, is the last resort. With open massage and internal defibrillation, it may be possible to resuscitate a heart that has been refractory to other efforts. However, if it is used, it should be done after no more than 15 to 20 minutes of unsuccessful effort.

Following successful resuscitation, the patient should be given ventilatory support, cardiac monitoring should be established, and a central venous or pulmonary artery catheter should be inserted. The patient should be managed as if he had cardiogenic shock. Aftercare may be considerably more difficult than initial resuscitation.

• • •

In summary, CPR is an essential body of techniques for any practitioner. Although only a physician can carry out advanced cardiac life support, the techniques of basic life support should be mastered by all medical professionals.

15

Principles of trauma care

The survival of patients with multiple injuries is largely dependent on the time interval from injury to definitive care. This interval has been termed the "golden hour," and it represents that period in which prompt diagnosis and initial therapy can save the most lives.

To improve trauma care, the American College of Surgeons has developed the *Acute Trauma Life Support* course, devoted to the principles of rapid initial assessment, life-saving interventions, stabilization and possible transfer. This course is augmented by a similar course on pre-hospital trauma care sponsored by the National Association of Emergency Medical Technicians.

The purpose of this chapter is not to create trauma experts. However, every practitioner should know the principles of trauma care.

ATLS is based on a prioritized approach. There are four phases. First, a *primary survey* is done to identify life-threatening conditions such as airway obstruction and shock. Simultaneous management of these conditions is begun. Next, *resuscitation* is carried out. Third, a *secondary survey* consisting of a detailed examination of the patient is made to identify all problems. Finally, *definitive care* of all injuries is planned and carried out.

INITIAL ASSESSMENT—THE PRIMARY SURVEY

In dealing with the severely injured, it is vitally important to recognize and treat immediately life-threatening states that can be managed by relatively simple surgical techniques. To ensure thoroughness and proper sequence of therapy, treatment priorities and protocols have been established: **A-B-C-D-E.**

A Airway maintenance with C-spine control

The first priority in any trauma patient is the maintenance of a patent airway. A diagnosis of real or impending airway obstruction should be presumed if there is an altered level of consciousness, either agitation (hypoxia) or obtundation (hypercarbia), or trauma to the head, face, or neck.

Before attempting any manipulation of the airway, consider the possibility of a cervical spine injury. This should be ruled out by an adequate x-ray examination showing all seven cervical vertebra. Until then, proceed with great caution. Immobilize the head, maintain in-line cervical traction, and avoid hyperextension. Cervical spine fracture must be suspected in any patient with injuries above the clavicle, especially major head injuries.

Basic maneuvers in clearing the airway include the jaw thrust and chin lift techniques (Fig. 13-1). The chin lift is the technique of choice. If used properly, it will not result in hyperextension of the neck. Blood and secretions should be removed with a rigid suction tip.

To protect the airway in a patient with spontaneous respirations, an oropharyngeal or nasopharyngeal airway should be considered (Chapter 13). The nasopharyngeal airway is better tolerated by the conscious patient.

If the patient is not breathing adequately, endotracheal intubation must be performed. If cervical spine injury is suspected, nasotracheal intubation is preferred. However, the orotracheal tube is indicated in the apneic patient. If intubation is necessary in patients with suspected or known cervical spine injury, use in-line cervical traction to prevent hyperextension.

Inability to intubate the trachea is the primary indication for cricothyroidotomy (Chapter 13). Jet insufflation or cricothyroidotomy should also be considered if severe maxillofacial trauma or suspected cervical spine injury precludes orotracheal intubation.

B Breathing

Once the airway has been secured, the practitioner should direct his attention to the mechanics of breathing. Several thoracic injuries can prove rapidly lethal because of the effect on cardiorespiratory physiology, yet their treatment is often accomplished by simple surgical techniques. The practitioner should be familiar with the symptoms of tension pneumothorax, open pneumothorax, massive hemothorax, flail chest and cardiac tamponade.

A *tension pneumothorax* is caused by a "one-way" valve, between the lung, or outside, and the pleural cavity. Air enters the pleural cavity with each inspiration but is not expelled on respiration. In time, air under pressure will fill the pleural cavity, thereby collapsing the lungs and inhibiting blood flow to the heart.

The diagnostic signs of tension pneumothorax include respiratory distress, tracheal deviation, unilateral absence of breath sounds with hyperresonance, and hypotension with distended neck veins. Immediate therapy consists simply of the rapid insertion of a large caliber needle into the pleural space (via the second intercostal space in the midclavicular line). Definitive therapy is tube thoracostomy, as outlined in Chapter 10.

An *open pneumothorax*, or sucking chest wound, causes hypoventilation and hypoxia because, with inspiration, outside air enters the pleural cavity, and the lung fails to expand. Open pneumothorax is best treated, initially, by an occlusive dressing taped securely over the wound on three sides only. This flap allows for the escape of air during inspiration. A chest tube should be placed as soon as possible (Chapter 10).

A *massive hemothorax* can cause cardiorespiratory embarrassment by collapsing the lung and also by blood loss. It should be treated by tube thoracostomy (Chapter 10).

Flail chest causes respiratory embarrassment in two ways. First, a segment of chest wall has lost bony continuity and moves paradoxically with inspiration and expiration. Second, there is contusion of the underlying lung. Initial therapy consists of airway control, administration of oxygen, and volume replacement. If this is not sufficient, or if there are numerous flail segments, endotracheal intubation and assisted ventilation using a volume cycled respirator is indicated.

Cardiac tamponade may lead to death rapidly, since as it does not take much blood within the pericardial sac to impede ventricular filling and thus cardiac output. The classic findings of cardiac tamponade are hypotension in the face of an elevated venous pressure, muffled heart tones, and pulsus paradoxus. Pericardiocentesis, as outlined in Chapter 10, may be life-saving but is only temporary. Tamponade eventually requires open thoracotomy as soon as possible.

After treating or ruling out the above life-threatening thoracic injuries, the practitioner should now direct his attention to maintaining the circulation and controlling blood loss.

C Circulation (shock and hemorrhage)

The prime objective is to restore and maintain an adequate circulating blood volume. The physiologic response of the patient indicates the amount of blood lost.

Class I hemorrhage (15% of blood volume, or 750 ml in the average adult)

This amount of blood loss produces minimal symptoms and may be managed by crystalloid infusion.

Class II hemorrhage (15% to 30% of blood volume, or 750 to 1500 ml)

Despite the loss of one liter (or 1000 ml) of blood, the clinical findings are minimal. Blood pressure is usually maintained. A decrease in pulse pressure and mild tachycardia, approximately 100 beats/min, is noted. There is slowed capillary refill. At this stage the patient exhibits only mild anxiety and the urine output is usually below 30 ml/hr.

Class III hemorrhage (30% to 40% blood volume, or 1500 to 2000 ml)

This is the stage at which hypovolemia manifests itself as hypotension. The patient has tachycardia (>120 beats/min.), and both blood pressure and pulse pressure are decreased. The respiratory rate is 30 to 40/min. The patient is anxious and usually confused. The urinary output is markedly decreased.

Class IV hemorrhage (more than 40% blood volume, or over 2000 ml)

This stage of hemorrhage is life-threatening and requires immediate resuscitation. The blood pressure is markedly decreased. The patient has a tachycardia (>140) and is markedly tachypneic. The patient is confused and lethargic. Urinary output is negligible.

Management of hemorrhage

The length and severity of hypotension with consequent hypoperfusion plays a significant role in the overall outcome of trauma. The practitioner should restore the circulating blood volume as rapidly as possible and control any bleeding.

Restoration of circulating blood volume is of prime importance. Venous access must be obtained rapidly, as outlined in Chapter 7. At least 2 lines must be secured with large-bore cannulas—at least 16 gauge. As these lines are placed, blood should be obtained for type and crossmatch or type and screen, depending on the urgency. Screened type specific blood can usually be obtained in 10 to 15 minutes and may be used in the emergency situation.

The initial resuscitation fluid is lactated Ringer's, given at 30 to 35 ml/kg (2 L in the average adult) as a bolus. When calculating the amount of crystalloid necessary for complete resuscitation, keep in mind that 300 ml of crystalloid should be given for each 100 ml of blood lost. If the patient is not adequately resuscitated after the infusion of 3 to 4 L of crystalloid, then blood, or at least colloid, should be added to the regimen. Crystalloid is usually sufficient to restore circulating volume in Class I and II hemorrhage. Blood is almost always needed in Class III and IV. Non-crossmatched Type O negative blood is often needed in Class IV with ongoing hemorrhage.

Correlation of the physiologic state of the patient with the time interval from trauma to arrival gives the practitioner a guideline not only of the amount of blood lost, but also of the rate at which hemorrhage is occurring. It also allows a methodical approach to restoration and maintenance of blood volume.

An important corollary to fluid resuscitation is the control of external hemorrhage to prevent or diminish ongoing blood loss. Control of external hemorrhage is best achieved by either direct pressure or pressure dressings. Tourniquets and hemostatic clamps are contraindicated. Immobilization of any fractures will help reduce continued blood loss.

The use of the PASG (pneumatic antishock garment) has become very popular in prehospital care. The practitioner should look upon this device as an artificial means of supporting perfusion pressure. It should not interfere with the primary goal of obtaining an adequate circulatory volume. Every attempt should be made to develop and maintain an adequate perfusion pressure without the necessity for PASG. When normal perfusion pressures are obtained, the PASG is slowly deflated. The abdominal portion is deflated first, followed by each leg. If a fall in blood pressure is noted, deflation is stopped and a further increment of fluid is given.

It is not always appropriate to apply a blood pressure cuff because initial assessment should be performed as rapidly as possible. The practitioner can rely on peripheral pulses. A carotid pulse is palpable at 60 mm Hg. A radial pulse indicates a systolic pressure of at least 80 mm Hg.

D Disability (brief neurologic examination)

After resuscitation has been initiated, a cursory neurological exam is performed. The level of consciousness is determined using the AVPU method.

A = Alert
V = Responsive to Vocal stimuli
P = Responsive to Painful stimuli
U = Unresponsive

Pupillary size and reactivity should also be noted at this time.

E Exposure

At this point the patient should be completely exposed in preparation to the more detailed secondary survey. Before proceeding with this survey, however, one should reevaluate the patient's response to previously instituted resuscitation and begin other modalities of resuscitation.

Supplemental oxygen, if not needed earlier, should be started at this time. Two large-caliber intravenous lines should be secured and ECG monitoring should be initiated. A nasogastric tube should be placed if there is no evidence of possible cribiform plate fracture (if such a fracture is present, the nasogastric tube may enter the cranial vault).

A urinary catheter should also be placed if there is no suggestion of urethral disruption: for example, blood at the meatus, scrotal hematoma, or high-riding prostrate upon rectal examination.

Once these measures are complete and the continued adequacy of resuscitative efforts has been validated, attention is directed to a more complete examination.

SECONDARY SURVEY

A complete systemic examination is next. Begin with an examination of the head with careful scrutiny of the eyes. Reevaluate pupil size and reactivity, look for fundal and conjunctival hemorrhages and lens dislocation. The head should be thoroughly examined for evidence of maxillofacial or cranial fractures. Patients with maxillofacial injury should be treated as if they have a cervical spine fracture until x-ray films showing all seven cervical vertebrae have been obtained.

In examination of the neck, close attention should be given to the position of the trachea, evidence of hematoma or subcutaneous air, and the status of the neck veins. Penetrating injuries through the platysma should be noted but not explored at this time.

On reexamination of the chest, pay particular attention to chest wall movement, presence of paradoxical motion, and pattern of breathing. Complete palpation of the chest, including each rib and the clavicles, should suggest the presence of rib fractures. Careful auscultation may suggest the possibility of either lung contusion or intrapleural air or blood.

Abdominal injury is often difficult to diagnose and slow to evolve, so that repeated examinations are often necessary. The hallmark of abdominal injury is pain. In association with unexplained blood loss, pain is often sufficient to surgically explore the abdomen. Peritoneal lavage is indicated in patients with a neurologic injury or an impaired sensorium and should be considered in the presence of equivocal findings. Peritoneal lavage is contraindicated if there is evidence of prior abdominal surgery and should be performed only after the urinary bladder has been emptied.

A rectal examination is essential. Particular attention should be given to the integrity of the rectal wall, the position of the prostate, and the presence of blood.

Examine the patient for skeletal injury. Contusions and deformities are noted and long bones, as well as the pelvis, are carefully examined. Necessary splints should be applied and appropriate x-ray films obtained. A more complete neurologic exam is now obtained along with an **AMPLE** past history.

Allergies
Medications
Past illness
Last meal
Events

DEFINITIVE CARE

The primary and secondary survey, along with the initiation of life-saving care, should be completed in approximately 20 minutes. The patient is now ready for definitive care or transfer. The practitioner should continue to monitor and reevaluate the patient until definitive care is initiated or transport is instituted.

• • •

The rapid assessment of the trauma victim with the prompt initiation of life-saving interventions is extremely important for a successful outcome. This chapter briefly outlines the principles involved in the initial assessment and stabilization. Practitioners who deal with trauma are urged to increase their skills by taking the Acute Trauma Life Support course.

Index

Page numbers in *italics* indicate illustrations.
Page numbers followed by *t* indicate tables.

226 *Index*

O

Orotracheal intubation, 186, 188-192
Over-needle catheters for venipuncture, technique for, 110-112
Overdose of anesthetic agent, 63-64
Oxygen in airway management, 202

P

Packing in abscess management, 99-100
Paracentesis, 163-166
Parenteral nutrition, long-term, long-term central venous access for, 119-122
Paronychia, surgical drainage of, 103
PDS sutures, 30
Peel-away sheath, catheter placement with, for long-term central venous access, 122
Penicillin(s)
  for cellulitis, 98
  semisynthetic, in abscess management, 99
  for staphylococcal wound infections, 104
Percutaneous suprapubiccystomy, 177-178
Pericardial cavity, drainage of, 162-163
Pericardiocentesis, 162-163
Peripheral venipuncture, techniques for, 105-112
Perirectal abscess, surgical drainage of, 103
Peritoneal cavity, drainage of, 163-170
Peritoneal lavage, 167-170
Pharyngeal airway, 186, 187
Phenylephrine for hypotension from anesthetic overdose, 64
pHisoHex in skin preparation, 3
Pilonidal cysts, surgical drainage of, 104
Pleural cavity, drainage of, 150-162
  chest tube in, 152-162
  thoracentesis in, 150-152
Pneumothorax
  complicating tracheostomy, 198
  open, in thoracic trauma, 214
  tension, in thoracic trauma, 214
Polydioxanone sutures, 30
Polyester sutures, 30

Polyglactin 910 sutures, 28, 30
Polyglycolic acid sutures, 28, 30
Polypropylene monofilament sutures, 31
Popoff sutures, needles for, 35
Pressor agents, systemic, in advanced life support, 210-211
Pressure measurements, central venous, 112-119; *see also* Central venous access, techniques for
Procainamide in advanced life support, 209
Procaine as anesthetic agent, 62
Prophylaxis, tetanus, for acute wounds, 88-89
Pulmonary artery catheter, techniques for placement of, 130-132
Pulmonary capillary wedge pressure (PCWP), measurement of, catheter placement for, 130-132
Punch biopsy, techniques for, 145-146
Puncture
  arterial, techniques for, 133-135
  lumbar, 170-172

R

Rabies immune globulin for animal bites, 91
Rabies vaccination for animal bites, 89, 90-91
Radial artery
  cutdown techniques for, 138-142
  puncture of, techniques for, 133, 134
Rake retractor, 22, 23
Rectal examination in trauma care, 218
Red cell count in peritoneal lavage, 169-170
Regional intravenous block, 71-72
Resuscitation, cardiopulmonary, 203-211; *see* Cardiopulmonary resuscitation
Retractors, 21-23
Ring forceps, 21
Robinson forceps for nasotracheal intubation, 193